SEX FOR THE THIRD AGE

Patricia Maris

A book for improving the lives of couples, divorcees and single men and women over 45, bringing awareness to new ways to live the best part of the best years of their lives.

enigma7™

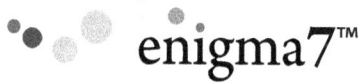

1st Edition Published by enigma7™

ISBN 978-1-925419-07-8

Patricia Maris and Alan Gold
Design Steven Cook Creative

www.enigma7.com.au
patriciam@enigma7.com.au

Ross Porter, thank you for always believing in and encouraging me, I will always treasure your friendship.

And as for you my dearest Alan Gold, without you this book would have never become possible. Thank you for teaching me the craft of creative writing. I promise I will get better with every book.

Much love to both of you.

Ms P

To the reader, please note that in this book, at certain points, you see a code like this:

It will direct you to a website where you'll see further information extending the ideas we're discussing at that point.

If you haven't already downloaded the free QR Code scanner app all you have to do is download one from the app store or Google play, just search 'QR Code Scanner'. Once downloaded you will be able to use your tablet or smartphone device to scan any code you see throughout this book.

In Health and Wellness

Patricia Maris

SEX
FOR THE
THIRD
AGE

This is a book about sex. Not Hollywood sex, or the sex which young people think is exclusively theirs, but sex for older people.

AN INTRODUCTION

Sex for the Third Age is about intimate
sex and sexual intimacy for men and
women who have entered their Third Age.

But what is this magical Third Age, when
does it occur and what does it mean?

There are three ages into which most human lives can be defined.
We'll come to the first and Second Ages soon, but let's define the
Third Age. That's when couples have grown to a stage in their lives
when their children are independent when they're probably empty-
nesters, or when they're divorced and living separately or when
they're at a stage in their lives when intimacy has taken second or
third place in the scheme of what's important. People who reach
their Third Age may be married or divorced, widows or widowers,
single, separated, or in a transient relationship.

But to have reached their Third Age, men and women will have
grown and developed to the point where they're anticipating the
joys of comfort, security and the ability to relax from their life's
work of raising a family and succeeding in a career.

And the Third Age is that time in their lives when possibly for
the first time they have space and freedom to unwind and revisit
the physical joys of sexual intimacy with a partner of their choice.
No more kids demanding their attention, no more struggling up the
corporate ladder, no more worrying about bills, this is the Age of
reflection and resting on laurels. This is the age where the thrills of
sex can begin again.

But this isn't just a book about the physical aspect of sex for
more mature men and women. There are many books, videos, and
guides for men and women who have put aside those earlier mind-
blowing sexual adventures because of the demands of kids, work
and responsibilities. No, this is about something allied, but different
from sex. This is a book about intimacy.

Intimacy. That's what sex should always be about. Intimacy is so often missing in today's world of instant sexual encounters, of Facebook and Twitter, and especially of the ubiquitous pornography which suffuses the internet.

Pornography is about the functionality of sex; it's about eroticism, extremism, and orgasm. Pornography and intimacy are at opposite ends of the pendulum's swing.

In this book, we're dealing with intimacy in its full meaning. All the tools of physical sexuality, pornography, sex toys, and mastering the art of physical sex can be part of the road which leads to intimacy, but at the end of this path, for full and complete enjoyment and fulfilment, intimacy has to be reached. It's not a signpost on the way to a climax it's the reason for the journey. Without intimacy, sex will always lead to physical satisfaction, but like a takeaway meal; you'll be starving for more after a couple of hours. But if intimacy is reached, the feelings, satisfactions and well-being will be sublimated, and the memory will linger far longer than the fulfilment.

So let's begin with a few definitions to help you decide whether this is the book for you. Let's start with the title *Sex for the Third Age*.

What is the Third Age? There are three ages in people's lives. Each age has its joys and frustrations, but of the three, no age has more potential for human happiness, yet is more prone to frustration, than the Third Age.

There are no fixed chronological divisions for the ages. The First Age can last until the age of 16 or the age of 26; the Second Age can come to an end at 45 or 65, and the Third Age can begin when the kids leave home, or when people retire and gain freedom from the daily grind of working.

The First Age ends when young people have the first of a series of sexual and emotional relationships. This is the age of young people learning and coming to terms with themselves as sexual beings. It's the age when youngsters hold hands, kiss, and experience what they consider to be love for the first time. This is an age which is training for their next stage. This stage is a permanent relationship in which a home, a family and an asset base are created. This stage can last for ten, twenty or more years. This is an age of consolidation.

And then, when the children grow and begin to live independent lives, the couple enters their Third Age. This age is where the couples have built a family, security, and now they ready themselves for the rest of their lives together.

Of course, huge generalisations have been made in this thumbnail sketch, because many people live lives as gay singles or couples, as permanent heterosexual singles, or in a series of de facto relationships ... but the Second Age is one of consolidation in their personal, professional and social lives.

But even when we're dealing with a married couple, there are many exceptions to this idyllic scenario. For a start, fifty percent of all marriages in the Western World end in divorce; those couples which don't separate often stay together in a state of emotional and physical neutrality, where much of the passion which brought them together is believed to be no longer a part of their relationship. Why? Partly because of the pressures of work and the increasing levels of debt and family responsibility, men and women often become isolated within their relationship ... isolated from their wives or husbands or partners. There may be a social and emotional relationship, but the driving force, which brought them together, and which nurtured one and the other in the early and middle days of their relationship will have evaporated.

Gone are the loving cuddles, the hugs in bed, the long hours of fondling and feeling, the sharing of sexual dreams and fantasies, requirements and aspirations.

And yet, unlike the days of our parents and grandparents, men and women are no longer dying as they enter this Third Age, as better health and nutrition allows us to live far beyond our three score years and ten. And let's reiterate the shocking reality that half of all marriages in the West end in divorce and acrimony, which leads to anger and alienation, withdrawal and emotional and sexual frustration.

But assuming that the couple stays together, and they enter this third golden age of peace, serenity and loving companionship, one thing happens which casts a shadow over the culmination of their hopes and dreams. In most cases, intimacy is no long a part of the relationship. Sex may happen once or twice a week or month but loving, caring affection is usually absent.

Of course, it's infinitely worse for widows and widowers, divorcees or those who are suddenly single for reasons which are many and varied. In these cases, single people have to rely on sexual fantasies or, at worst, sexual sublimation, to get through their nights. The Internet and its oceans of pornography are now providing cold sexual release, but not fulfilment or happiness, too many single men and women; and increasingly to many married men and women who masturbate in front of a computer in another room while their partner is asleep.

But whatever the reason, sexual abstinence from a partner is a cause of frustration, depression, high blood pressure, hormonal imbalance, headaches, emotional eating and much more which lead to obesity and a plague of other problems.

Sex for the Third Age is a guide to making this third golden age of people's lives into the most exquisite and beautiful time they have.

So the Third Age is the age where we start to reflect on the life we've lived, and must not … ever be considered as the beginning of the journey, which leads to the end of the road. Rather, the Third Age is that blissful time in our lives when we can enjoy all that we have worked so hard to achieve, and we have the memories, the knowledge, the experience and the reflective abilities to know both where we're going, and avoiding the roadblocks along the way. Think of those great advertisements for retirement homes, where a middle-aged man and woman gaze into the distance, which is full of oceans and golf courses and a cloudless sky. The reality of retirement homes is of course often painfully different, but this book is about making the Third Age more into the advertisement than the nursing home.

OK, we've dealt with what defines the Third Age. Now we have to understand what we mean by 'Intimacy'. Intimacy doesn't have to be between married men and women or men and men or women and women. Intimacy doesn't depend on our legal status as husband or wife, partner or *de facto*, significant other or casual lover. Intimacy is beyond gender, beyond colour, beyond race, beyond age.

Intimacy is a state of YOUR mind. It doesn't even depend on a relationship. You can be intimate with a stranger.

Let's repeat that for a moment ... you can experience intimacy with a stranger.

Yes, that seems counter-intuitive and strangely contradictory to accepted norms, but it's true. Intimacy isn't about your wife, partner or lover. Intimacy is about YOU. It's about dropping the walls and barriers you've built up around yourself which prevent you, yes YOU ... from being in touch with your inner self. It prevents you from being free to express the intimacy that is still misunderstood (and often ridiculed) in our society.

More and more today, with the ubiquity of sex on television, the Internet and even advertisements, intimacy is increasingly marginalised and derided by the industry of the quick orgasm, by those who believe that sex is a transient and frequent expedition into climax and release. The idea of a long, tender, sharing, caring and transparent experience of intimacy between lovers has become so marginalised through all-pervasive media that we no longer even consider it part of a sexual tryst. Even when we masturbate, when we fantasise and think erotically, we're burdened by guilt. We do it secretly behind a closed door; we stop instantly and cover ourselves when we hear somebody approach.

So ... Why the distance between sex and intimacy, the paradox between satisfaction and guilt? Let's for a moment look at the situation of sexual congress between two people. Let's imagine, just for this example, of a man going into a brothel. He pays his money; he goes into a room, and a prostitute comes to him and services his needs. He climaxes and leaves.

Has any intimacy occurred? No, obviously not. Because the man was there to buy a woman's time (and body) for an hour; and she was there to sell her body and time to him in exchange for money.

There was little which resulted in the exchange other than sexual release. Because when the man's time and money ran out, the prostitute immediately withdrew her services without consideration of his feelings.

Now let's look at the same man (or woman) who goes into a bar or a club, and starts to converse with a stranger. There's a mutual attraction. There's a thrilling sensation. There's the look, the suggestion, the proposition, the excitement. They go to a room (his, hers, a hotel this is a fantasy remember, so let's just assume that they go somewhere) and they lay together. The fantasy that began in the bar continues into the bedroom.

Is there intimacy in this situation? You bet! Why? Because the man and woman (or man and man or woman and woman) don't have inhibitions. They want each other, and they drop their barriers. They probably whisper intimate things into each other's ear. They are free to talk about their fears and hopes, their fantasies and aspirations. They will expose themselves, one to the other, and not just because of their naked bodies.

And it's more much more than the fact that there is no money exchanged or judgment in the second illustration. It's because they've met and are fulfilling a desire, which initially is hormonal, but later becomes driven by dropping their inhibitions and opening themselves up to intimacy.

Ok, this might seem contrary to norms and, as we've just said, counter-intuitive. After all, most of us require weeks or months in a relationship before we'll be entirely sexual. But much of that timeline is because we expect certain behaviour in others we expect our future partners to be monogamous, we expect them to be faithful, to chose us as the one, and close their minds, hearts and bodies to others who might be rivals. There is an assumption in society that norms will be adhered to; a preconception of how committed partners will behave one to the other.

This is a reflection of our parental upbringing. It's what most of us observed in our parents, and we grew up in a household where lovers, boyfriends, girlfriends and alternative relationships between our parents and others were never discussed. In most of our homes, monogamy was the norm. And that's what our parents saw in their homes when they were growing up with our grandparents and so on backwards through the ages.

And this silence, this assumption that some things were never disclosed or discussed, created barriers in our minds about acceptable behaviour, opening ourselves up to others, and feeling that intimacy should only be between ourselves and the most significant person in our lives at that time.

In the First Age and indeed the Second Age, these barriers are a necessary and protective mechanism for the welfare of ourselves and our partners and children. Without those obstacles, which prevent us looking and lusting after others, society would be a mess. We need parameters, which confine intimacy between significant partners.

Of course, in Western society, fifty percent ... yes, half ... of all marriages divorce. But this is little to do with intimacy. In the majority of cases, it's because society (read religion) has determined that adultery is utterly unacceptable in a loving relationship and is a reason to split the partners asunder.

Many happy and fruitful marriages, even those with profound and abiding intimacy, are riddled with a secret, furtive adulterous relationships conducted outside of the marital house. Husbands go to conferences and play around; wives do the same. Partners wander secretly to a neighbours' house and have furtive sex; businesspeople do it with assistants, married people do it with other men or women. It happens consistently, and it is rarely a reflection on the love or intimacy between the couple.

And it might have many reasons the husband or the wife is exhausted and incapable of the preferred sexual response the husband or wife might have become too familiar, and the partner is desirous of relieving the sexual excitement which once was there, but is now absent. The reasons for adultery are manifold and timeless. But that doesn't mean, not for one moment, that there's a deficit of intimacy between the couple when they make love.

A man or a woman can return from an intimate sexual encounter with another partner with another, and feel joy at seeing his permanent partner, in making love to him or her ... and in many cases identified by researchers into this field ... there's often a greatly heightened sexual relationship between partners when one of them has strayed furtively and had an alternative sexual experience.

So welcome to *Sex for the Third Age*. As we said at the beginning of this introduction, *Sex for the Third Age* is about intimate sex and sexual intimacy for men and women who have entered their Third Age. And as we detail how intimacy is so intimately tied up with well-being, nutrition, breathing, hydration, movement, thinking, will-power and rest, so we'll see how the Third Age isn't the beginning of the end of our lives, but the beginning of the most exciting, uncomplicated, enjoyable, fulfilling, momentous and sexy time we've ever had the pleasure of experiencing.

CHAPTER ONE

Why people in their Third Age put sex at the bottom of their life's agenda ...

AND JUST WHAT PART DOES INTIMACY PLAY?

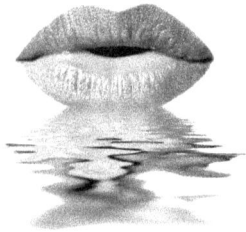

"Intimacy begins with oneself. It does no good to try to find intimacy with friends, lovers and family if you are starting out from alienation and division within yourself."

Thomas Moore

Sex for the Third Age is about the intimacy of sex for people who have time in their lives for the time of their lives. It is all about intimacy, and what makes us intimate. It's both about the interior ability to allow ourselves to be intimate to lower the barriers and allow intimacy to be a part of the relationship we want to develop with a partner and it's about the outside factors, which will help us become intimate.

We'll come on to the seven foundational pillars of wellness without which intimacy can't gain a foothold in our conscious lives. In brief, these have been created to become a lifestyle in which intimacy can reside. They're all about nutrition, exercise, breathing, hydration, rest, willpower, thoughts and movement, and each has been created as a module to lead you simply and cautiously into better health and a more relaxed and positive state of mind. And the very best way of reaching intimacy in the Third Age is through this 'reconstitution' of your mind and body. As you proceed through this book, step by cautious step, we'll lead you gently but positively into a better 'YOU', but for now, let's deal with a definition so that we're completely transparent about what we're going to be achieving.

And that definition is the term 'intimacy'.

Intimacy doesn't depend on how long a couple has been together or even the circumstances of their relationship. As the Author Jane Austen wrote in her book, *Sense and Sensibility*, "It is not time or opportunity that is to determine intimacy – it is disposition alone. Seven years would be insufficient to make some people acquainted with each other, and seven days are more than enough for others".

Intimacy means different things to different people, and at different times of our lives. Most fortunate children have an intimate relationship with their mothers and fathers. Its based on trust, empathy and understanding. It begins with breastfeeding and continues all the way through holding hands as we cross a road. The intimacy between child and parent is bound up in security and safety, or so it should be, as we don't live in a perfect world, and tragically many children grow up without knowing any better, and hence don't learn it. Intimacy should, by rights, exist between parents and children; it is incumbent on parents to create an ideal world for their children in which intimacy is a natural part of childhood.

Teens often have intimate relationships with their 'BFF' ... best friend forever ... until one of them says something unkind, and then the love turns to hatred, which turns to love again when there's a tearful apology. Newlyweds have intimate relationships with each other, but more often it's based on physical sex than emotional intensity.

And so on through the ages of men and women. And we can be intimate with our closest friends; with our counsellors with priests and teachers all of these caring and sharing relationships are built on intimacy.

And while we're talking about the different ages and stages of intimacy, especially sexual intimacy, let's make a strenuous point here, and that's the often-disparaging and disrespectful attitude of the young to the sexuality and intimacy of men and women in their Third Age. There's an ageist attitude held by the young that sex, sexuality and intimacy belongs to them; that as far as their parents or grandparents are concerned, the older you get, the less right you have to sex and intimacy.

There is an old joke about a daughter recently enamoured of a new boyfriend, who asks her mother, "Have you ever been in love, I mean *really* in love ... not like you are with Dad ...?"

Young people don't believe (or can't cope with) the idea that older mature people engage in physical sex. They think that sex between people of an older generation is dirty, shameful, disgusting or plain wrong. There's the assumption that older people are sexually inadequate, or do it by rote, or are unadventurous or routine, or that even if they do indulge in sex, it's purely mechanical. They seem to think that active, romantic, and erotic sex is a preserve of the young and that an older person's interest in eroticism, sexuality and desire is contrary to the Laws of Nature. We owe it to our younger generation, the respect to teach them how to cut their own cloth to fit the suit of age, and so they can show us the respect that we have organically earned.

Anybody who gets sexually turned on and is above the age of 50 knows that this attitude says more about the young than it does about men and women in their Third Age because interest in sex doesn't diminish with age. It may be sublimated, or diverted, constrained or conditioned, but it's still there, as virile and active as it was when they were young and brash.

So what is 'Intimacy'?

Let's start off by accepting that the desire for intimacy doesn't diminish with age, and should never be limited by the constraints of societal norms. So intimacy can be experienced between hetero and homosexual couples, by transgender and bi-sexual couples; it doesn't have to conform to the limits or labels of what society determines. But the ability to be physically intimate can be affected by heath disorders, the inevitable emotional upheavals which are hormone-driven in older people, natural ageing, and the inevitable vicissitudes that life throws in our paths, such as divorce, death, drugs and disruption.

But that's the desire for intimacy. It doesn't answer what intimacy is. Perhaps the best way of understanding the meaning of intimacy is to try to define it not constraining it within the boundaries of words, but to create a platform so that we all know what we're discussing. Because if you think that sex is intimacy, then you're going to miss out on much of what this book has to offer. Sex is great, but as we'll soon see, sexual intimacy is the purest form of communication and enjoyment.

Intimacy is having a tender, open, honest relationship with another person in which transparency between you is the natural order; it's where the deepest thoughts and feelings and desires can be expressed openly and honestly without fear of retribution; it's where you give and are given, the sense of worth, value, understanding and endorsement which each of you requires as the true nature of your relationship. And that shared value is a validation of the emotional, physical and intellectual merits which you put into the relationship. Once that platform is established, once the transparency is achieved, then the more you're willing to share, and allow to be shared by your partner, the greater and more intense will be the depth of intimacy you'll reach.

Intimacy is about closeness, and it takes both courage and practice for somebody, especially someone who's usually reticent, to allow another to be that close. But we're close to ourselves when we desire isolation and privacy when we seek solitude to be alone with our thoughts. And we can learn to lower the barriers we've built up inside ourselves to allow ourselves to be close to us, especially those with whom we desire to be intimate.

Because of such closeness, such connection and sharing, is a reflection of our deepest and most secluded world, the inner sanctum which we have learned to protect from the view or influence of others.

This leads to the most astounding realisation about intimacy that intimacy is about YOU ... about lowering your barriers and allowing others in. Intimacy starts from your inside, from your inner being. And that means being utterly honest with the person with whom you want to be intimate in a way, which you've probably never done before, because of your fear of rejection or alienation.

We learn these concerns from childhood when a sibling or a teacher or a friend ridicules us when we reveal something about ourselves. We soon learn that telling or revealing passions is something, which can lead to our being hurt, and so we build up walls which prevent our revealing those things which we now hold within us, and which we rarely allow the outside world to see.

In essence, we need to create, and willingly share a clear space within ourselves and then invite somebody to share that space with us. All of this must be undertaken with mutual respect and care and consideration for another. We must learn to listen, to understand and to empathise. The biggest problem we will have in creating this space is by truly understanding what intimacy means to us. If this doesn't happen, then it will be nearly impossible to swim in the warm and willing waters of intimacy.

That's why communication is the heart of intimacy, the very essence of sharing. Intimacy is all about a revelation of desire, about opening up, about communicating and revealing. It's about talking and sharing and communicating deeply held yearnings and longings and desires and trusting that the partner with whom you want to be intimate, would accept your needs and requirements and be willing and able to share in them. And it's about listening to your partner and allowing that same sharing from him or her.

Always remember that intimacy is a two-way street. Just as you must learn to be transparent and communicative, so you must learn the art and power of listening and understanding the needs of your partner. If you don't, intimacy won't last longer than a single occasion.

So it should be obvious that intimacy is very different from physical sex. Sex can be nothing more than a physical function carried out without joy, sharing, communication, intimacy or compassion. Or, if it's entered with joy and passion, communication and intimacy, it can be utterly breathtakingly monumentally wonderful, and this is regardless of whether we're young, middle-aged or elderly. When sex is truly intimate, and when intimacy leads to physical sex, there are few greater moments in our lives, which are as profound and well, intimate.

And so how do we apply intimacy. How do you facilitate conversations with your partner so that you can learn to become intimate? Because intimacy is as much about learning how to be intimate, as it is in being intimate; and this can change with each partner. You can develop a deep and abide intimacy with one partner in a matter of a day or more, yet with another partner, that intimacy might take weeks or even months to develop, if at all.

Learning how to be intimate in a relationship is learning how to communicate. And that can begin with talking with yourself. It can be a question and answer session, working out the best way of introducing the desire or craving which could lead to intimacy. It all comes back to communication.

And there are many ways of communicating. Let's create a scenario, which may have little or nothing to do with you and your needs, but which is illustrative of how to proceed to be intimate with a partner.

Let's just imagine that you have a particular yearning for your partner to wear black underwear. You know that if you suggest it over breakfast, your partner will look at you as though you'd just had a sudden brain- explosion, or you'd been reading some article that wasn't appropriate to cereal, eggs and bacon. Any suggestion about what underwear you'd like your partner to wear, made at an inappropriate time or place, will usually have a negative effect. And there is a better way of doing it.

How? Well, you have to learn how to communicate your desire and need in a way, which creates a platform for mutual respect and understanding. Go out shopping with your partner, and by gentle guidance, find yourself in the lingerie section of a department store. Make a suggestion that your partner would look lovely in some new underwear, and suggest that black might suit her. If she looks at you in surprise, then admit that you'd love to see her in black lingerie by being in a safe environment of a public place like lingerie outlet, any embarrassment will be muted by the surroundings, and this could very well work in your favour.

But what if your sexual turn-on and craving for the intimate contact that is missing from you life is, shall we say, a more unusual? Say, for instance that you want to be spanked while you're making love. Instead of asking, which might create shock and aversion in your partner's reaction, simply buy or hire a DVD, which you know contains a spanking scene, and when it happens, judge your partner's reaction when you say that it turns you on. Then have a frank, open, honest, intimate and transparent discussion about the fact that you've always wanted to be spanked.

No, these aren't fetishes which only the depraved and degenerate want to enjoy ... these, and a hundred other likes and desires are part of the sexual makeup of all of us, and only by being honest in communicating our desires, are we going to be able to reach the depth of intimacy which is our right, as human beings, and especially in our Third Age.

One of my clients is a retired prostitute, a lady who needed my lifestyle and wellness coaching in getting her life back on track after years in the sex industry. She was often asked by clients to indulge them in sexual fetishes which they were either too embarrassed to discuss with their wives and partners, or had been rebuffed.

Here's what she told me ...

"Because most clients are so ashamed of desires within themselves they view as unnatural, or which their partners won't allow them to indulge in, they hide them and they remain unexplored. Most prostitutes are so keen to see the next client for his money that they don't bother to explore and find out. In marketing, there's the 80-20 rule, where 80% of business comes from 20% of clients. I learned this early on, and worked my heart out to satisfy a client, allowing him to explore his fantasies.

"Few of us, who might be turned on by the sight of shapely legs or round and curvaceous breasts or a tight and muscular backside, can envisage the different numbers of fetishes that are out there. I made a list of the different fetishes I've come across, or been asked to involve myself with over my long career as a whore. Here are some of them ... just a few of the A's and B's, but there's an entire alphabet of fetishes which men and women would love to explore if they could ... anal, bananas, breast implants, bending over, big beautiful women, beads, big breasts, bikinis, bisexuality, biting, blindfolds, bondage, boots, bottles, business suits ..."

She was wonderfully honest, and it really goes to show the vast range of desires which men and women usually have to sublimate. And isn't this, after all, one of the main reasons why partners leave the marital bed and go out to seek another.

Isn't this the reason for affairs ... because we're too constrained to express our deeply held desires with our partners, and so we live a life akin to Keat's Knight in *La Belle Dame Sans Merci* ... alone and palely loitering.

Familiarity and this inability to communicate so often causes men and women to be alone and frustrated in their relationships that they go and pay for sex in a brothel, or they actively seek a partner outside of the permanent relationship they've developed. Yet if they were open and honest and transparent in their communication, if they had the ability to express their desires, if they told their partners what it was that they needed for a full and active sexual and intimate life, then affairs would be unnecessary in their relationship it might not happen to them in the same way as it would happen to others.

And of course, we've said that it's a two-way street, because you have to create a platform for your partner to be able to express his or her desires openly and honestly, so that you're not guessing or despairing that you're intimate life is in the doldrums, but you have the ability to discuss what your partner needs and wants.

So we've now come to terms with the nature and concept of Intimacy. From childhood, we either learn the joys of intimacy, or we're shut out from it and fail to live our lives in the full bloom of intimacy. We become survivors and not participants.

And so often, this continues throughout our lives, even as we enter the Third Age. So why are older people, who usually have the time and resources, incapable of showing and experiencing intimacy?

Out of all experiences, one of the most intimate experiences we can have with other people is through sex. Yes, it's intimate and naturally close well, very very close ... but it doesn't necessarily equate to intimacy. To be intimate in our Third Age, we must learn, train ourselves and practice to regain this foundation of humanity by applying some of the principles we've mentioned above.

But is there a practical way of learning to be intimate? Well, in most instances, provided the internal barriers are lowered (it's too difficult to drop them simply ... we're always too reserved to do an 180-degree turn), and then we can become increasingly intimate.

We could start by verbalising our hopes and desires. Telling our partner how we'd like to pleasure them and invite them into our fantasy world; sharing our dreams and feelings, and what we'd like to do if our partners gave us free rein. And perhaps reading this chapter of this book together, so that both you and your partner can share in these thoughts.

Once you've spoken at length and honestly about your desires and those things you'd like to do to your partner, then at a later stage, ask your partner what he/she would like to do to you. Assure your partner that whatever they suggest will be considered by you seriously, non-judgmentally and honestly.

You may agree, or you may disagree, but so long as you're open to suggestions and discuss your likes and dislikes in an adult and non-prejudicial way, you and your partner have opened a line of communication.

Now, from a practical perspective, this is the time to allow space between desire and fulfilment. This is the time to back off, and allow your suggestions to your partner, and his/hers to you, to sink in. And the next time you indulge in sexual intimacy, this is the time to whisper in your partner's ear about your and his/her desires.

Continue the conversation but in a light-hearted and non-disparaging fashion. Suggest a visit to a shop or the purchase of a movie or a way of extending the love making session so that it becomes the fulfilment of desire, rather than a threat that one-day will be realised.

These are just some of the suggestions, which can be made to open up a dialogue, communication. But what's the purpose of this conversation? It's to breach the walls, which prevent intimacy! It's to lower the barricades; it's to come to terms with the reality that intimacy is YOUR issue, and that if you accept that lack of intimacy is often the situation which YOU bring to the relationship, then you're well on your way to being intimate and changing the way you treat yourself and relate to your partner.

And for those in our Third Age, it's the dawning of a whole, new, wonderful and sunny day.

CHAPTER TWO

When you lose your appetite for sex
1+1=3

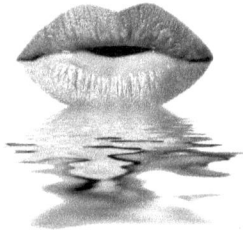

"The starting point of all achievement is desire."

Napoleon Hill

In the previous chapter, we covered aspects of affection, understanding and tenderness, and the primacy of being intimate as a foundation for truly beautiful, enjoyable and teeth-clenching sex, especially for men and women who have reached their Third Age.

In older years, men and women might find physical exercise a bit of a strain, and once-enjoyable gardening might cause muscular and joint pains these days unlike twenty or thirty years ago. But sex is the one time of which our bodies always seem to rise to the occasion.

Ok, so we might not swing from the lampshades like when we were teens, and maybe we're not as sexually experimental or energetic as once we were. But the enjoyment we get from sex, as we grow older, is undiminished and easily the equivalent of those sweaty, timeless days when we began to explore another person's body.

And it's the delight and gratification we find in sex, which is paramount, the sharing and closeness, rather than the race to a scream-laden orgasm. Just because sex no longer lasts for hours, the minutes spent in intimate congress with our partners now that we're in our Third Age are as blissful as they were when we were younger. The intensity of our enjoyment of sex in our third period doesn't depend on athleticism, vigour or suppleness, but on the willingness of each of us to share, care, nurture, and attend to the needs, wants, desires, hopes and cravings of our partners.

There's a key algorithm for sex, which applies to any stage of life, but it seems that we truly understand it when we reach our Third Age. It's a simple mathematical equation, the concept of synergy.

$$1 + 1 = 3$$

It signifies that you and your partner are greater than the sum of each other. When you come together in intimate sex, there's a synergy between you, which exceeds the sum of its parts, the two of you, in the most intimate and sharing congress. It's almost as if, by reaching this state of intimacy, just the two of you in a private moment you've become elevated into a level beyond normal. It's as though the world isn't a part of you anymore and you're not a part of the world, but you exist in a realm, which is otherworldly.

No, it's not a spiritual, magical, religious or non-corporeal concept, it's practical and realistic, because, in the intimacy of sexual understanding and sharing, you grow in more ways than just the physical. Or so it should be; unfortunately, after having trained our brains with little or no time to have sex due to other aspects of life, we have grown to understand that's all it is and never question what could be improved. After all, we don't know what we don't know!

But even the most intimate and loving couples often have a multitude of issues when it comes to sex. Boredom, sameness, lack of time, lack of sexual adventure, exhaustion, diet, health and other problems often intervene. And the longer we've been with the same partner, the less we're inclined to seek out the freshness in them, which is often a driving force in sex.

The men and women who come to me with issues of sexual incompatibility, inability or simple boredom, have often been together for a long time, and are seeking a simple solution. It's one of the reasons we search for a new partner, or enter into an affair, or go to professional sex workers. We're seeking freshness to sexuality, newness, daring, and an adventure, which we're not finding in our partners. There's nothing more exciting than a new partner, more titillating; more exhilarating. But this is nothing more than an unwillingness to connect at an intimate level with a long-term partner.

Wouldn't it be better perhaps to discover something new about our spouse, wife, or husband as we grow older together instead of looking for 'IT' elsewhere? What if we could change the perception and that with some improved communication and a little effort and health on our side we can keep the torch of sensual love alive within our chosen relationship? Just as Tango was a dance made for two, so is the 'Horizontal Tango'. Yes two willing and enamoured people who love each other unconditionally working together to make this work, even in the bedroom.

Unfortunately, this does not ring true for a lot of couples and instead what we tend to do with our partners, especially our long-term partners, often try to find a reason, or in some cases, an excuse for the lack of sex. We talk about the decline in hormones as a cause for sexual incapability, or stress as a joy-killer, or health issues such as heart or other bodily functions as the reason we're no longer operating as we once were.

In the case of men, they use excuses like job stress, exhaustion, or erectile dysfunction as the reason they're not making love as often as they once did. But if they turned their focus to the 'synergy', the intimacy, the joy and togetherness of sex, rather than the ACT of sex itself, which should be the very core of the relationship, then things would flow naturally. Perhaps if women, rather than only daydreaming about what they want from their partners could verbalise their feelings and talk about their needs, their wants, their desires, what works and what doesn't. We were born naked, hungry, crying, and alone. Some of us got over these hurdles and learnt through life by making mistakes and experimenting, some of us listened to our older brothers or sisters for guidance. But one thing is absolute; none of us was given a manual the moment the Doctor or midwife cut the umbilical cord. It is and always will be up to us to do what is best for ourselves.

Often, it's the 'expectation' of mind-numbing sex, which is what causes the disappointment and lack of physical ability in men, or physical response in women. Once I explain to men, women, or couples who come to see me that sex, especially in the Third Age, is more about sharing and caring than of a sexual release, the reaction is often startling. It's almost as if they are released from the treadmill of expectation, and can just be casual and enjoy little moments of sharing and caring, of real intimacy, without any expectations of reaching orgasm. The remarkable thing is that once that hope is removed from the equation, with tenderness and caring, a climax is often reached.

It's the self-fulfilling prediction of what should be, rather than what could be, which is what so often causes disappointment, incapacity or inadequacy in the mutual intimacy between couples. When sex just becomes the concentration on the performance, and not on the sharing and caring for each other without any expectations, performance issues take over leading to disappointment and frustration.

In any age, from teens to senility, we need to be kind to ourselves, and not consider our performance as some medal-winning athletic competition. Especially in our Third Age, when stresses and strains can have a dangerous and deleterious impact on our bodily functions, we must remember that it's the intimacy, which is more important than the climax, the journey rather than the destination. That's not to underestimate the importance of a strong orgasm, but rather to enter into an intimate moment with the intention of enjoying the intimacy for itself, the closeness, the sharing, rather than breaking the tape at the end of the race with the crowds cheering our performance.

Over the years, I've treated many men and women who thought that there was a physical or emotional problem stopping them from having enjoyable sex.

One of the first things I do is to relieve them of the pressure by just telling them that sex can be fulfilling and satisfying even if there is no penetration, even if there is no orgasm. The important thing is to enter into an intimate occasion with not a single expectation. To just go with the flow, enjoy each other's bodies and each other's energy. Only then, in time, with patience, love and understanding, an orgasm will result and let's face it, very few penises work on command. So stop telling yourselves, "it won't work!" instead, understand that some stay soft even when the man desperately desires an erection and in that case what you must do is to fantasise and play a visual game of what once turned you on, as there is no right or wrong in fantasising and drawing stimuli from your imagination.

But let's get one thing clear. Regardless of your preconceptions, and irrespective of the demands of society, intimacy doesn't depend on sex. And sex doesn't depend on affection. Intimacy is a contact sport for the soul and sex is only one aspect of the game. So let's take this 'game' metaphor a bit further. Players accumulate experiences the more they practice and play their sports. If you play and train alone, you'll learn some of the rules that work for you, but you won't properly appreciate all that the game has to offer. Once you start playing and training with a team, you'll soon learn the art of testing the rules, bending them a bit, sharing interactive experiences and making up new rules to suit yourselves. You never stop learning, because as the game develops, so will you and the rest of your team. You also need to keep training and playing to maintain freshness and keep up your level of fitness so that you don't lose your strength and ability to play the game. This analogy rings true for intimacy as pushing and testing your limitations and boundaries with a partner is a whole new experience than just understanding yourself within your limits.

You can live a life without an orgasm, although you would be missing out. Unless of course, if a person is asexual – the definition of Asexuality is the lack of sexual attraction to anyone or low or absent interest in or desire for sexual practice. In some societies, young people can have the most intimate of sexual experiences while abstaining from almost all physical encounters. Indeed, the traditional sexual practice for many women who get married as virgins in southern Europe where family and societal constraints prevent physical relationships can be incredibly intimate, even leading to private sexual completion, without doing more than holding hands. It can be in words, in a glance, in the way in which a body moves. It's suggestion, rather than reality, and it goes to prove that the greatest sexual organ is between your ears, and yes you guessed it, this applies to both men and women alike.

The key to achieving and maintaining an intimate and ultimately fulfilling life is to find the fuel that suits YOU. It's the one fuel that not only ignites intimacy but helps keep you going and that is trust.

Trust is an ambiguous concept, but it needs to be understood if we are going to allow intimacy, whether it be self-intimacy or intimacy with others, into our lives.

Let's go back a bit and talk about a man and a woman who come together wanting to begin a relationship. He comes to that relationship full of expectations and hopes. But he also comes with a set of rules and regulations, which he has adopted throughout his childhood and in later life experiences. He has fears and complexities. He wants to be open and trusting, but so much in his life prevents him from being completely free.

She comes with the same sets of baggage. Her mother, father, sisters and brothers, teachers, priests and friends have built in past behaviours, which will govern her acceptance and her behaviour with this new man when they begin their relationship.

So our couple goes out on a date, and there is a strong physical attraction. They plan to meet again, and at the end of their rendezvous, there is the first kiss, the first feeling, the first attempts at physicality.

All good so far but in subsequent meetings when he says something, or she does something, their baggage, this being emotional, physical, spiritual and mental baggage will begin to intervene and barriers will start to grow between and around them.

Sure, most couples can overcome their baggage and accept the new parameters because the desire for sexual intimacy, fellowship or friendship will enable them to close their eyes to those things which they don't particularly like in their prospective partner.

So where does intimacy come in? Where does trust come in?

Let's assume that the couple loves each other and decide to marry. During the first few years, their honeymoon period, they manage to put their baggage to one side, because of their joy in their relationship and their desire to make it work.

However, once the routine has set in when regularity becomes the norm, then even though they are adults, the voice of their inner child will become increasingly insistent. The voice of their inner child wants to regain the cosy feeling of intimacy, which was there in their first flirty meetings. But as the couple become used to each other, and the bond they have created becomes more formal than emotional, the baggage they have managed to subsume until now starts to come to the fore, and the voice of the inner child becomes louder and louder in attempts to be heard.

Soon the couple starts to rely on the precepts of personal history rather than the reality of their current circumstance. And the statements they make to each other tend to become increasingly like a couple of lawyers in a courtroom.

The inner child, confused, abused and frightened becomes more and more alarmed. Trust is fractured, sides are taken, and they become like two boxers in opposite corners, summing each other up, testing each other's mettle. This reminds me of the Burning man sculpture. This Love sculpture features two wire adult figures sitting back-to-back. Representing – to me – the accumulation of fears and baggage we carry throughout our lives. Inside their frames stand two infants who are reaching out to one another. I have interpreted this as the chemistry, love, innocence and security, which we all seek as human beings. For us mammals, it is in our basic DNA to need a physical human connection. As the sun sets and the moon rises, the two unspoilt infant figures light up and set the surrounding area aglow. I would refer to this as the honeymoon stage of the relationship; the stunning contrast between the wire and this illumination makes me think that it is always going to be possible to reconnect with the most important part of us. All we need is to free that inner child and be open to it. Once we achieve that, we can reconnect with others and be open hence, emotionally available.

You see, I know that it doesn't matter how independent and strong-willed we think we are, I can say for certain that every once in a while, you get an unexplainable yearning just to be held, comforted and told, 'Everything is going to be OK'.

This appetite for love does not make you, in any way, weak. The world, and often your parents – especially if you are a boy – may tell you to 'toughen up', that 'the only person you need is yourself', and 'Don't show your feelings'. Well, I've got news for you, as soon as we become conscious of existence the principle of duality at once confronts us; thus where there is an action, there is going to be a reaction. And if you suppress your feelings one day eventually they will burst out in a mixture of ways, both emotionally and physically they will be exposed. When we act in opposition to our feelings, it causes internal stress. When this becomes chronic stress, the tense reaction of our muscles, which in fact accumulates that stress and causes inflammation, leads to irritation and subsequently if left untreated might cause infection, which leads to illness. At a later age all those symptoms might show what is now call Autoimmune disorders and here is what Mr. Google has to say about them.

"Autoimmune diseases are a broad range of related diseases in which a person's immune system produces an inappropriate response against its own cells, tissues and/or organs, resulting in inflammation and damage. There are over 80 different autoimmune diseases, and these range from common to very rare diseases".

Doctors know these symptoms and recognise that syndrome all too well, in kids, they've even created a whole range of initials for them – *ACH*, ADD, ADHD – the list goes on and on ...

We need to be surrounded by people. Like the lyrics to the 1964 song *People* sung by Barbra Streisand:

> *People, people who need people are the*
> *luckiest people in the world.*

When we become adults, we begin to complicate the first youthful and innocent relationships with our misconceptions, influenced perceptions, emotional limitation, and 50% of the time, our parallel lives. Unfortunately, this only consumes the relationship; it destroys the fuel, which once ignited the trust we had in each other, and it all comes down to a lack of communication. Building communication skills at an intimate level is paramount, feeling free to acquire the tools to be able to express feelings, needs, desires and hopes, without the judgment of a partner. If we don't, then this, 50% of the time, in which we live a parallel life, will lead to divorce. But divorce doesn't only have to be dealing with husband and wife; these days, more and more people are in casual, de facto relationships, and so separation can be as costly, damaging and enervating to couples as it can be to a married one. 50% is the current rate of divorced couples in the Western world.

I think that a couple of real life instances will explain better than philosophical words what all of this means.

A couple came to consult with me because of intense guilt feelings about an intimate sexual experience they'd both had. Their religious upbringings were the very antithesis of what this middle-aged couple had recently done, and now the wife was sick to the stomach. It was tough for them, to even go to Church, or even see her elderly parents; ashamed that their activity was ruining her life, and so they sought out to talk the situation through with a life coach, me.

One day, the husband was at an airport waiting to fly home when he phoned his wife. It had been a long couple of days of business meetings and loneliness in a hotel room, and so when he called his wife to chat, something in him broke. As he was talking to her, she asked him, jokingly, whether he'd been a good man in the hotel, or whether he'd had fun with another woman in his room.

He was surprised, as his wife never spoke like this. It seemed that she had missed his company, and so her fantasies were coming to the fore. So he played along. Even though he was in a crowded airport, he found a corner where he could have a private conversation and continued to speak to her. He asked her if she was sure she wanted to hear, and she said that she was certain; that she was alone in their bedroom, laying on their bed, and would love to hear his misadventures.

So he told her that yes, he'd had a woman from the business meeting stay with him for dinner, and they'd had a bit too much wine, and so she'd come to his room, and they had made love. He often had these fantasies, but sublimated them and had never spoken about them in public, and certainly not to his wife.

To his complete shock, she interrupted, and said that while he'd been away, she had two men come to their house to fix the plumbing. In the bathroom, she had looked at their bodies, had admired the line, which showed just above their trousers as they bent over to fix a pipe. She had put her hand where their cracks were and felt inside their pants. They'd immediately turned and stripped her of her skirt, panties, top and bra, and taken her into the bedroom, where they had f**ked her.

She told him how she had experienced orgasm after orgasm, and then she asked her husband whether he'd like to hear the rest of the story. Still amazed by what his wife had said, he asked her "Are you into phone sex? After all these years I had no idea".

She responded in a new found husky dark tone, "Darling, stay with me. I want to continue. I want to be all you need".

So he embellished and continued, "Don't think that this woman who stayed with me was alone", he said. "She called up her sister who was also staying with her and came up to my room. Her sister was just as riled and ready to go as we were and they were amazing". He asked his wife "Do you want me to tell you what they did to me?" "Was it what the plumbers did to me?" his wife responded. "Yes, both working on different parts of my body at the same time ..."

So the conversation continued on the phone until his plane was announced, and they had to stop their phone fantasies. The flight home was excruciating, he couldn't stop thinking about their conversation, in the taxi, and when he walked through his front door, he couldn't wait to get home and see his wife.

His wife, demure and unassuming, was in the kitchen finishing off the preparations for their dinner. He kissed her and asked how she was. They exchanged pleasantries until, over the dinner, he asked, "I was stunned by our conversation on the phone when I was waiting at the airport. I never knew –"

"That wasn't me", she interrupted, her face flushing a deep red.

He frowned and asked what she meant by that remark.

She gulped and murmured, almost as a whisper even though they were alone in the house, "I don't know what came over me. I'd had an afternoon nap, and you woke me up, and I just spoke like a slut ... a whore, I'm so ashamed of my behaviour! I don't want you ever to mention it again. Is that clear?"

But he argued. He said that if that was a fantasy, then they had to bring it out into the open. She reacted as if she had been caught out in a lie, and she insisted that they drop the conversation.

That's the way it continued for six weeks, he trying to open up the conversation, and she shutting it down before it had even begun. Eventually, after endless severe and hateful quarrels, a friend of theirs referred them to me.

That's when, as a life coach and an objective 3rd party, I created a neutral landscape for them to open up in, to truly open up. I talked about trust; that she had to trust me, as did he; and that they had to trust each other sufficiently to air their differences. He wanted to explore their fantasies; she wanted to bury them under a rock. We needed to find a middle ground, a point of difference that would take both their needs and desires into consideration without one of them having to give up something that they held so precious.

The principal of 1+1 = 3 requires some give and take, it does not mean losing yourself, and acceptance is paramount in this case.

So I spoke to them and introduced them to the idea of their innocent child which has been buried deeply inside the adults that they had become. I told them that they were victims of their upbringing. At first, she objected to the word 'victim'. She said she'd had a great childhood. However, as we began to examine how strictly her parents had brought her up, how she'd been forbidden alcohol until she was 18, how she'd been chaperoned on dates by an older sister. Then she began to defend her parents; until she accepted that many of her vivid dreams had probably been the outpouring of frustration.

I asked her whether she'd masturbated much in her teens, and she'd denied it vehemently, but when I told her that I had masturbated from my early teens, and still did so when I was alone and frustrated, she became silent. Slowly, softly and cautiously she began admitting that yes, occasionally, she would play with herself.

And then it was like her dam had burst. She laughed, and then smiled, and then became a bit teary, and then laughed again; and her innocent child suddenly appeared through the cracks. She admitted that she'd masturbated regularly as a girl, and had felt ashamed of her actions and that when her husband was away, she had powerful sexual feelings and desires.

Her husband stayed silent for much of the time, looking down at the floor. I was pleased, because this wasn't a moment for his intervention, and he seemed to understand that. She was talking to me, just me, and it was more of a priestly confessional than anything.

How did it end up? Well, they went away, and returned seven times to see me; (one session for each of the pillars I use in my program to help my clients find balance in their consumed lives) each time, they told me of the fantasies they had discussed. All of them were safe and pleasant. But did they ever turn these fantasies into a reality? Well, that's their business.

Now let me tell you about another couple who came to see me some time ago. This couple exemplifies what happens when sex, and especially intimacy, disappears from a marriage and how it can, in fact, be restored.

I've changed their names to protect their privacy. John was a middle-aged middle-ranking executive who had worked for the same supermarket chain since he had left school.

His wife, Margaret was a former airline stewardess whom he had met on a business trip when they were staying in the same hotel. It was lust, rather than love, at first sight. And the desire remained between them for the first couple of years, until the arrival of their first child.

He was given a promotional appointment, but it was contingent to another city, which meant that Margaret had to move home and away from her family. Although Margaret was happy for John, the move brought a real crisis to their marriage and caused unending disaffection between them. A once happy and contented couple started to find disappointment in each other.

The disappointment migrated from the lounge room and the kitchen into the bedroom. Suddenly the lust, which had been a large part of the reason they came together initially, was no longer a part of the relationship intimacy.

After two years of living away from John and Margaret's home base, and seven years of marriage, they started to discuss divorce. Both had lost the love and lust they had felt for each other at the beginning of their relationship.

But sense prevailed, and because of their young daughter, they decided to stay together until the little girl was old enough to understand. Sex as relief was still a part of their relationship, and Margaret soon found herself accidentally pregnant. John swears to this day that he took precautions, but Margaret soon found herself blaming him for the unexpected arrival of their second child that was now growing inside her womb.

After another two years of a less-than-happy marriage, and with two young children at home, Margaret longed for the sound of John getting into his car and driving to work. She had put the kids into daycare and would go shopping or meet friends for coffee or lunch. It didn't bother her that this was another source of John's disaffection with her. She accepted his barbs about her laziness and in effect told him to suck it up.

And then she met Rudi, a German-born merchant banker living in her city. He was having lunch in a crowded restaurant, and she was shown to his table, the last seat in the house. They smiled, and talked about things in general, and then she asked him whether or not he was married. She didn't mean any sexual overtones, and he was smart and sophisticated enough to realise that she was making conversation. He told her that he was separated from his wife and that the marriage was, in effect, over.

Margaret empathised, and told him the condition of her relationship with John. There followed a moment of silence, until he said, casually, "I've finished my meal. Now's the time when I should pay the bill and leave".

She nodded.

And he continued, "But if I stay until you've finished your meal, and then we have a coffee together, I'm going to take it as a sign that you'll want to meet me again. Is that a fair assessment?"

She looked at him long and hard and nodded.

A couple of days later, they were in bed, and Margaret enjoyed the same level and depth and intensity of sex that she had in her early days with John.

It took her four months before she flung her affair with Rudi in John's face, and blamed him and his coldness towards her for forcing her to seek satisfaction elsewhere. John told her that enough was enough, and said that they should separate and go to lawyers.

The attorney that Margaret found and confided in is a good friend of mine, and knowing the emotional and financial costs of the divorce, and also recognising the devastation it would have on the two children, he urged her and John to consult me.

As soon as they did, I identified a couple whose communication was absent and whose intimacy was non-existent. The easiest thing to do would be to allow the two to separate and leave it to somebody else to pick up the pieces. That's not the way I operate, as a wellness expert, I knew that if I could just get them to communicate, to understand what the other was saying ... to hear the meaning behind the words, only then there was a possibility that the marriage could be rescued. And four lives wouldn't be damaged.

The moment they sat in my office, I could see from their body language that the gulf between them was broad and profound. Folded arms, bodies twisted just far enough away from each other that John and Margaret could only see each other out of the corner of their eyes, mouths were drawn tightly so that any possibility of a smile had become little more than a grimace.

I began the conversation with them by asking a simple question of each of them. "John, what first attracted you to Margaret, what was it that made you feel dizzy at the thought of seeing her again and again? And Margaret, what was it about John that made a beautiful woman like yourself decide that he was the man you wanted to spend the rest of your life with?"

Initially, they both shrugged and said that they simply couldn't remember. John stated he knew she was attractive, but that was all.

So I took them back to their first meeting, then their first date, and asked the questions a second time. John smiled and admitted that it was Margaret's breasts, which first appealed to him. "... they were tantalising, and the way she wore her dress made her very seductive". I asked whether he still found them perky and attractive, and he admitted that "Yes, they were one of the features of her that I still enjoy looking at".

Margaret admitted that it was John's smile, and the masculine way he wore his suit, that first attracted her to him and his friendly demeanour.

Half an hour into the session, they were both talking about the good points, both physical and emotional about the other. The ice had been broken, and they were speaking in gentler terms about the reasons for their attraction in the early stages of their relationship.

So I sent them both home with some homework until we saw each other again the following week. It was simple, and I knew that they would find it initially demeaning, but it was an important step for breaking the ice, which was freezing their marriage and stultifying their relationship. I told them each to get a simple notepad and divide the pages into two vertical sections. The left-hand side was of the things, which their partner had done during the week which had shown kindness and consideration. The right-hand side of the page was of the things the partner had done which had been unfair, unkind, and thoughtless.

I knew just what would happen, and a week later, I was proven right. John's list was three pages of complaints with just a line or two dealing with Margaret's consideration. The complaints were universally petty and trivial, such as staying too long in the bathroom, not tidying the house for his arrival from work, and arranging for friends to come around at night when she knew he would be exhausted after a day at work.

Margaret's list was nowhere near as long as John's but was dealing with much bigger problems; not helping to get the kids ready for school, not earning enough to allow her the freedom she wanted from housework, not wanting to go overseas on holiday.

Upon this revelation, I deliberately read out John's list to Margaret, and then Margaret's to John. At first, each wore a look of self-justification, feeling vindicated in their analysis. But as I read through the lists, I could see how uncomfortable each was about the things they'd said about the other.

It didn't take long for both John and Margaret to understand that the cause of much of each one's disaffection with the other was not just petty, but it was a lack of communication. And without communication, as we saw in the previous chapter, intimacy can't flourish.

After three more hour-long sessions, they were both sufficiently relaxed in my presence, and with each other, for me to suggest how to reignite the intimacy they once experienced back into their lives.

For their next set of homework, I suggested that they write down their most intimate thoughts about what each would like to do with the other. I told them to be as explicit, as transparent, and as open as they possibly could be. And I assured them that the list wouldn't be disclosed to the other partner.

The following week, I discovered that Margaret's list was full of aspirations; that John would be more of a husband and a partner than he'd been for the past five or more years. And John's list was aspirational concerning sexuality. His list included sexy lingerie, secret liaisons in public places, watching adult movies together.

I surprised them both by telling them to pick one from their list, and to organise babysitting for the children, then over a dinner in a restaurant to openly and gently tell each other what their greatest desire was. And they did. It was the first time, in a long time that they had felt relaxed in each other's company. They laughed, they talked, they even held hands.

It took two more similar sessions before I could entice them to have sexual contact with each other. But I advised them not to go all the way, but instead to touch, to fondle, to kiss and cuddle, and to re-learn what it was that had initially attracted them to each other.

EMOTIONAL CURRENCY

"There are three wishes of every man: to be healthy, to be rich by honest means, and to be beautiful". – Plato

So what's the common denominator that people, especially women, bring into the lives of a couple and which lasts until the Third Age? Women are born with a bank account, and that account is labelled 'Beauty'.

As we grow older, this bank account evolves into a different form of beauty. A beauty that isn't defined by Playboy or Penthouse or Woman's Weekly or what society defines beauty, as one of its mutable trends, but instead, 'beauty' is the eternal essence of womanhood. It's the charm, the outer and inner beauty, respect of self, self-possession and self-identity, which is part of them and which makes them women. It's the way they present themselves to the world, and it's their demeanour. It's the 'sense' appeal, as opposed to the 'sex' appeal by which men define women. Sure in their late teens and twenties it's the kind of beauty which perhaps will score them great sex when it comes to physical intimacy, but the long-lasting intimacy which will bring great sex needs to be nurtured as women advance into their mature, Third Age.

This same thing happens with men, as their hair thins, as their stomach forces them to add notches to their belts, as the once lush pubic hair starts to grey and become withered. Men look upon this as the maturity, which will attract MILFS (for the unworldly and those who don't visit pornography on the internet – you know you do! – a MILF is a 'mother I'd like to f**k'). Wrong! So wrong! Most men don't exude sexuality or ooze intimacy as they expand out of their trousers and slouch when they walk. They are not playboys anymore when they climb slowly upstairs or gasp when they have just run for the bus.

Men, just like women, have to consciously turn on their sexuality and intimacy buttons, and learn to find the comfort and inner being which women will find sexy and attractive, the one where women will yearn to be near to them, because of the gentle intimacy they'll find.

At every age, there will be better-looking people than us in the view of society, those who will attract the opposite sex like flies. Ok, so they're the lucky ones; and believe it or not, they're the ones who, as their beauty is no longer a part of their 'currency', need to increase their inner beauty, with age. They need to improve their charm, self-esteem, their personalities and that intrinsic pathway which will open them up to understanding and intimacy.

They are the ones who should be reading this book. They are the people who relied on their physical and not their inner beauty, to be complete women and men. Those of us who are not externally the type who might appear on a magazine cover learned as we left our parent's knees and wandered into a world of other people, that to be part of a group, we had to become attractive to that group. If external physicality didn't do it for us, then we had to quickly develop and accumulate the personal assets and forces which others found appealing.

Kindness, gentleness, consideration, generosity, empathy, sharing and caring are the very essence of intimacy, created by a regimen, which can be introduced at any time of your life. Regardless of your external beauty. You are not born with them; these are assets that you have to develop and accumulate in part from starting to socialise at kindergarten, then at school and then in the workforce but also from learning that your mind, brain and body are intimately linked.

So as we'll see in later chapters; Breathing, Rest, Exercise, Willpower, Hydration, Nutrition and the power of Positive Thinking, are all essential in creating the landscape in which intimacy becomes more than a part of your makeup. It is YOU.

CHAPTER THREE

Health problems and sexual activity

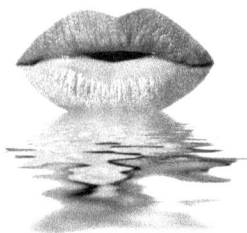

> *"Sex is the best cure. One good night of sex and your problems are gone."*
> Grace Jones

This chapter, in our incredible journey to bring back intimacy and sexuality for men and women in their Third Age deals with health challenges and the lack of sexual activity which is the bane of so many of our lives. As we say goodbye to our kids, lead a lonelier life as a divorcee, or try to come to terms with the fact that we are a widow or widower, we come to terms with the new-found idea that our sexual fulfilment which once made our lives so rich begins to evaporate.

Now that you've read the first two chapters, you'll understand that this doesn't have to be, and that much of the emptiness is because of questions around intimacy.

Many types of intimacy may or may not lead to sex. But life is more than sex, and sex is more than just the physical act. Without any doubt, intimacy will lead to a life, which is full, satisfying and exhilarating.

As opposed to a life which is little more than surviving and living one day to the next. So let's see what these different intimacies are and what they do for us.

INTELLECTUAL INTIMACY

This is without a doubt where it all starts if you have an intellectual, non-threatened cognitive connection with someone and you have no issues being in touch with your most inner self, chances are you will enjoy a more fulfilled and fulfilling relationship, either with a partner or with a friend. Any unproductive communication – or the need to be right – will tend towards the nullification of intimacy, leaving you to search for stimulation elsewhere. In order to deepen the bond between two people, you will need to be able to share simple things.

Things which don't have to be sexual or physically related, such as discussing a movie, a book, or a current affair issue, nurturing and exploring someone else's thoughts and sharing yours is really essential to growing as a couple, or simply for self-improvement, as this can only lead to gaining confidence and attracting the right people into your life.

EMOTIONAL INTIMACY

Being true to ourselves doesn't come easy in that a lot of people just want to be 'right' instead of being truthful to themselves. Feeling able to talk about your own emotions with someone is really hard for most people at the best of times; it requires a strong understanding of who we are within ourselves, and nobody likes to feel vulnerable, which causes us to put up barriers or guards especially early in the relationship.

For people who have already suffered termination or disruption of a previous relationship, this proves to be even more challenging.

We find ourselves at ease when we are in the arms of a person who makes us feel that no matter what, they accept us without judgment; on the other hand we need to be able to offer the same space to our loved ones so that they too feel safe to open up to us on an emotional level.

But be observant of your own patterns of behaviour as you must know that 'pleasing everyone' is not the right approach, a healthy relationship should not be about 'who do you want me to be' rather it's about 'this is who I am'.

If you believe that your life and your feelings count and that you matter, then you will need to go beyond your ego-self because emotional intimacy is best achieved when you drop all survival techniques – behavioural patterns – and let your heart of hearts be kind and free.

This isn't just psychological talk. There's an easy way to do it. Feelings are important and do matter; your feelings count. But for them to be validated you need to be in tune with those emotions and talk about them so why not make time on the weekend, say on a Sunday morning over breakfast; or if you aren't in a relationship ask a friend out and have the same conversation with them.

Why? Because for once, you're talking about yourself to somebody you can trust. It might seem sound or feel at first somewhat self-centered and egotistical, but the reality is that in this controlled environment you are putting yourself first and that's one of the aspects of a mature and adult relationship with your partner/friend.

Please note here that we are talking about raw emotions not the superficial kind of talk.

Here are some ideas to help you get that ball rolling. Something that he or she doesn't know about; It can be important or trivial, but getting into the habit of sharing these emotions with your loved one will create a safe space in which you both can grow.

At the beginning of any relationship it could be simple things, like sharing an activity such as cooking together and while you are doing such activities you can start-up a meaningful conversation while choosing or selecting the ingredients for the recipe; your likes and dislikes and you can both take note of what your partner/friend's taste and opinion are, ensuring that when you include or omit it them in the future, they know that you've been thinking of them; or in a more physically intimate relationship how about showering together and perhaps using a sponge and soap to gently wash their back or surprise them by washing their more intimate parts.

When we are emotionally close, we can share personal feelings because these are critical aspects of our lives and the more we get to know and open up to that person the more opportunities you will have to become 'best friends'. These are the minimum requirements that constitute what we call the perfect combination of physical and emotional intimacy the rest of the 'other types' of intimacy is just a bonus.

Scan here to learn more on how to *Bring Intimacy Back*

Emotional Intimacy is truly important; but what if you find it difficult to let yourself get too close due to bad past experiences? Perhaps you find it problematic to unwind and feel emotionally safe with people even when you have known them for a long time.

Well here are seven tips to enable you to feel relaxed in your intimate relationships:

1. Get physically-close bit-by-bit. Not too quickly, but ensure that your intimacy has a physical component, right at the beginning of the relationship. Even the feeling of a gentle kiss goodnight on the cheek can last all week. You see, the intention with which we do things is what actually counts, as it is not the way we touch people but the intention with which we use our hands to touch and caress people as this is what they perceive, and how they will react to that touch.

2. Trust yourself and know that you deserve emotional intimacy, as you can't receive what you can't or aren't prepared to give.

3. Learn the difference between physical and emotional intimacy and what they mean to you. We often learn a pattern or interpret something because we have observed it and sometimes it just doesn't resonate within us, there may be the act of performing a gesture; whether it be a kiss or a playful tickle, but there is not emotion or intent behind this action. It is simply a mechanical movement. Learning to differentiate between what works for you and what doesn't can make a world of difference to our partner's reactions.

4. Make small revelations to your partner. Just letting him or her in on a little secret of yours will create a bond, an intimate connection between you; and that will encourage your partner to open up as well.

5. Don't force intimacy. It's not a competition or performance. Everybody needs his/her own time to open up – in the meantime you can develop or explore other kinds of intimacy.

6. Be open to the prospect of intimacy. Don't limit the outcome by having expectations of what your partner should or shouldn't be doing. If it doesn't happen, as you want it to, then open up and discuss it. Be frank, but understanding. It is a two-way street, so treat it as such.

7. Finally and most importantly, take care of your health; Exercise, Nutrition, Hydration, Movement, Rest and the other aspects of the wellness program will make you feel good, in fact, they will make you feel terrific! They will also add to the intimacy you want to experience. If you feel great from within, nothing can spoil that feeling.

Ok, those are the seven excellent tips of intimacy. But right from the beginning, let's get one thing absolutely clear. You deserve intimacy.

Let's say that again you deserve 'IN-TO-ME-SEE'.

It's your right as a human being to dive deep into who you are. Unlike members of the animal kingdom, we don't have periods of the year when we're on heat and are ripe and ready for sexual intercourse. People like you and me are willing for intercourse all the while. That's both the beauty and the curse of being human. The intimacy in the monkey and ape kingdom doesn't only come through sex, but also through grooming, tenderness, stroking and touching.

And that's the way it was when you were young and experiencing your first sexual encounters. You thrilled at the scent, the touch, the frissons of experiencing the opposite – or the same – sex.

Then you developed into a permanent relationship, and now you're in the golden years of your life. Older, experienced, comfortable, self-assured.

But your sex life isn't what you always dreamed it would be. Come on, be honest, you could do with more sex and not just sex, but intimacy too, which is so much a part of your thoughts. When you were younger, you would get into bed with your partner, and hug, kiss, cuddle, fondle, touch, explore and well, you know the rest.

But now that you're in your golden years you and your partner go into the bedroom, strip off, put on your pyjamas, get into your own sides of the bed, pick up your book and read until you are drowsy. Admit it that is what you do, isn't it?

So before we broach what can and will happen to the intimacy you DESERVE in the Third Age, let's talk about the problems that many, actually *most* men in their Third Age are having at the moment. I say 'men' because women can hide these problems. Men can't, because to be physically intimate, you need to be able to gain an erection, and as erections become trickier as we age, due to illness, blood circulation, lack of fitness, and proper stimulation and much more, men tend to avoid intimacy, rather than admit they can't get it up anymore. The meaning of physical intimacy for most men starts and ends with sex, this is a myth we must restore, according to *HealthyPlace.com* 'Physical Intimacy includes both sensuous and sexual activity usually between two people and the sharing of reactions, thoughts, and emotions that are involved in these activities. My question to men reading this, and the women, of course, is 'What part of our sensuality and our emotions are so hard to grasp?' Sexual Intercourse is not the only expression of 'Physical Intimacy'.

Few men won't allow themselves to acknowledge that they have a problem, or admit it to their wives. Instead, they will search outside their marital bedroom for what I call the 'sneeze of an organ' or simply put a quick orgasm – just simple sex to prove to themselves that they can still 'perform'. Here is where my theory of B1 and B2 often arises, and that is not Bananas in Pyjamas. B1 often refers as Brain one aka the penis and Brain two aka the brain. Of course, there's nothing wrong with following either one, but the guilt and insecurities that this unwanted and often uncontrollable behaviour brings along with it is hurtful and honestly, unnecessary. Yes, I know there are some men who just won't care about this, and unfortunately, those are the ones who won't be reading this book. What we need is the confidence to tell our loved ones that we need some stimulation, maybe a threesome or perhaps to watch some porn together it could even be a voyeuristic fantasy. If we enter into our deepest desires together instead of denying them, then relationships would not only last longer, but we would be healthier, happier and better off for it. The ideal situation would have been to start the connection with these strong foundations, and this book is perhaps the perfect gift to breaking the ice for some of you who are embarking on the second or dare I say the third or fourth relationship. And for those of you that are in a long term relationship, take a deep breath, relax and just bring a copy of this book to your partner, perhaps highlight the things that are important to you and let them highlight what is important to them, then find a beautiful place and chat about it. But if one of you can't grasp the idea of how or where to start even after reading this book, please do not hesitate to book an appointment and come to see me.

But it's not only our physical bodies, which prevent us from gaining an erection. While it's true that sex starts with a powerful desire for an orgasm, our minds have to be in it. It is here when we need to be brutally honest with ourselves, And if you are in a second or subsequent relationship and you have come from a broken partnership and the painful emotional experiences which these produce, there are often conflicting emotions which come to the mind and the penis and the mind and the vagina.

In which case you owe it to yourself to allow the time necessary to heal, because the external desire will change in most cases, especially in our Third Age, but only when the internal desire is ready, by being more positive and getting the moral, emotional and understanding support from family and friends, or people from work, you will find that motivation to reconnect within your inner happiness once again. Let's face it, 50% of permanent relationships aren't stable at all, and rather end in divorce or separation, and frequently both partners are left bruised and battered. In men, there is often a complex psychological relationship with the subsequent partner to ensure it doesn't happen again. And that sometimes makes intimacy apprehensive and challenging. I call this an emotional wall.

Just read what the prestigious professional journal, *The International Journal of Impotence Research* has to say about erectile dysfunction:

"Sexuality is one aspect of the emotional and physical intimacy that men and women experience through their lives. In adulthood, the closest intimacy is accomplished by physical and sexual relationships. Older adults desire sexual intimacy when there are a partner and a health status that allows sexual relationships. Older individuals desire to love and enjoy sexual activity in relation to personal circumstances, and when health status allows them to experience close relationships, most often within marriage. Normal changes occur in the phases of the sexual cycle with ageing, mainly men needing more time and stimulation to achieve a complete erection".

And of course, it's the same with a woman, because older ladies enjoy being pampered and require longer foreplay than when they were young to get their juices flowing.

"The importance of sex in maintaining a good relationship in a couple persists with advancing age but is affected by sexual dysfunction (SD). Primary-care providers of older patients with SD can approach various medical problems with focus on modifiable risk factors, to contribute to improving sexual function with ageing". Data collected between 2001 and 2002 in 27 000 men and women aged 40–80, across 29 countries, revealed that 28% of men and 39% of women had at least one complaint with sexual function. On the other side of the coin, 72% of older men and women either don't have an issue with sex, or have chosen not to disclose this information, which is more than likely the case. We also need to consider that. Unfortunately, embarrassment is a seriously prevalent cause of burying this problem in the bedroom. And by not talking about it openly, the issue can and will often continue to grow in the minds of a loving couple.

Nearly half of the men sampled between 70 and 80 reported having intercourse during the year previous to the interview, as opposed to 21% of the women. And 17% men and 23% women in the sample said 'older people no longer want sex'. Raising awareness and helping people to reclaim their state of wellbeing can reduce this number. In wellness, I have found more often than not that what you don't know, you just don't know! Hence you won't ask and as the cliché goes, 'knowledge is power'.

68% of men and 60% of women who took part in this study were in favour of older people using medical treatments to help enjoy sexual activity. The prevalence of erectile dysfunction in men mainly increased with age. A lack of interest in sex and the inability to reach an orgasm are frequently inhibitors among women, but surprisingly these are not as dependent on ageing. There are much more prevalent hormonal and psychological issues for women. When clinical patients in contrast to community-based women are screened, the prevalence of female sexual dysfunction (FSD) is higher, and there is the greater association with age.

The bottom line is that wellness, in particular, your state of wellness, is multi-faceted. It is both the wellness of the body and the wellness of the mind. In other parts of this book, I deal with Nutrition, Willpower, Breathing, Rest, Hydration, Exercise and Positive Thinking; all of which are aspects of the wellness that we need in order to feel the depth, beauty and excitement of intimacy, and as I have outlined Intimacy is the precursor to good, swinging-from-the-lampshade kind of sex.

When we find a loving partner, somebody suitable with whom we can share our needs, wants and desires (as well as a biology) then there's no reason why we can't reach orgasm. If you're among a majority of divorcees seeking to re-engage in a partnership, yet you fear that a relationship might put too many expectations on you; or that you might just have to give up your independence and lose your autonomy, then the problem lies within YOU. Sorry, but it's your problem, and it has to be dealt with, but don't worry, because the solution isn't hard and you've come to the right place. I'm here to assist you. You see just about every single person has more or less his/her ideas of what a perfect relationship looks, feels and tastes like, and perhaps you are constantly 'on trial', testing one relationship after another, finding out your likes and dislikes, wants and needs. Or maybe you are in the early, or later, stages of marriage and you are in the habit of telling yourself that if you don't focus on the little issues, that they will just go away eventually. Unfortunately, this is not the case. These problems will only compound, and you will slowly build up resentment towards your spouse. What you need is a Wellness Coach.

As a Wellness Coach I help you to recognise your own dreams, to refocus on your own goals, I help you to move past challenges that are preventing you from achieving a state of peace within yourself, thereby improving your relationships, and not only the romantic ones but the one that is *numero uno* ... the one with yourself. And together we achieve this by developing your strengths and abilities. This is the start of putting yourself and your happiness above anyone or anything else.

In short, you need to be willing to open up to your vulnerability. Becoming aware and in tune with your frailty is the only way to bring balance into your life.

A good place to start is by writing down what real intimacy means to you because this will have a profound impact on your sexual performance.

What do I mean by that? No, don't write down how big your penis should be, or how you like a woman with small, youthful, perky breasts or whether or not you are the right 'shape' or weight or pretty enough to find your perfect man. I want you to write down the far-reaching nature of intimacy, of what it's like to kiss, to cuddle, to stroke. Write down where you like to be touched, what turns you on, where your desires lie.

One of the most common problems is that many men start sex off with a good, firm rock solid erection, but within minutes, or when you first enter your partner, it goes flabby and floppy, and you lose it then you apologise, retreating frustrated. Many don't even gain a firm enough erection to enter their partner's body. And many now take and depend on Viagra, Cialis or Levitra to overcome erectile dysfunction, and can happily maintain an erection for an hour or so.

But as a rule of thumb, the older a man becomes, the more flaccid his penis will be unless he takes the appropriate, positive steps to implementing a healthy lifestyle.

Women, on the other hand, can participate in sex with a penis, fingers, a dildo or any other sexual aid. They can genuinely enjoy it, or look bored throughout, or pretend to be turned on. But with a man, there's no pretence.

If it ain't there, it ain't happening, and there is not hiding it.

And that's where intimacy becomes the master, not the servant, of sex; because intimate sex doesn't depend on penetration, orgasm, intercourse or ejaculation. Intimacy is determined only by the respect, the affection, the mood, the intensity and the adoration between the partners. It's all about balance and trust. Remember we are talking about the Third Age here where we are growing older together. Younger couples must seek advice if sex is an issue for either party.

So let's now look at the barriers to sexual activity among older men and women. These can evolve over advancing years, the lowering levels of testosterone – the male sexual hormone – or a plethora of other factors, such as physical limitations; a large stomach, asthma, emphysema or other illnesses which diminish energetic activities, medical side effects, or even the diseases for which such side effects are an unfortunate consequent; high blood pressure, diabetes and prostate problems can all be the reason behind erectile dysfunction.

THE BATTLEGROUND

For many men yes, this is a generalised statement, but men are mainly the cause of these problems the bedroom has changed from a sharing loving playground, into a battleground.

Because of his all-too-frequent 'Round One' failure to reach an erection, or his 'Round Ten' inability to have an orgasm. And so he blames the bed, the television, his kids, work, his boss and often even his wife or the damage that the last relationship left on him. Most of my male clients blamed others, especially their partners, for reduced sexual activities, performances and failures to either consummate or complete.

Often, if the wife were in the consultation, she would look dejected, glance at the floor, or even shrug her shoulders slightly to convey to me that we both knew that her husband was not coping with the truth.

Can you imagine what this blame game can do to your self-esteem?

Occasionally the wife would intervene and say that the husband had been a pathetic lover for decades, which would cause turmoil in the consultation and I would have to intervene. But rarely did the partner accept that he or she was as much at fault as the other. This is, indeed, an individual battlefield.

Because if truth be told, it was both of them who were failing in their levels of intimacy. If a husband couldn't reach an erection, due to any of a dozen reasons, it was their partners responsibility to help, assist and work with the partner to find a way to satisfy his sexual gratification and if this wasn't physically or mentally possible they were there to provide the intimacy which would be the mainstay of the relationship for all time, the same is true for a women who was unable to climax.

But this isn't a 100% pass-fail scenario! Because it is incumbent on the partner who can't reach satisfaction to tell the other partner what he/she needs and wants to be satisfied? Perhaps it's gentle rubbing, grasping and fondling, maybe oral stimulation, or a gentle erotic massage, there are a hundred different ways of satisfying a human being not involving penetration and erotic sex.

Eroticism is entirely satisfactory on its own, without the need for an orgasm. Sure, a climax is great, but it's not mandatory nor even necessary. Indeed, there's a form of sex called Edging, Peaking or Surfing. These types of orgasm control techniques rely on stimulation, with a deliberate refusal to reach orgasm.

The refusal to climax can last for days and when it finally comes, so to speak, it's what I call a full body orgasmic experience. It is such an intense sensation. The wait is well worth it. I highly recommend testing it, try to tease one another for at least ten consecutive days. Flirt with each other, do little things and send each other sextexts. And then, on the 10th day ever so softly drive each other nuts in the bedroom and try to control the urge of cumming then when you are both surfing the edge of the orgasm release yourselves in one massive explosion.

So, an orgasm isn't the be-all and end-all of sex. It's a beautiful climax, but far from mandatory. Nor is penetration if you have an empathetic partner and an intimate relationship where caring and sharing takes the place of teeth clenching, knee bending, head twitching yeehah sex.

Many doctors specialise in the loss of erection. If a medical condition causes it, then you MUST see your doctor. But the principles of the wellness advice are in many instances the key to remedying any issues. In fact, most doctors, when you tell them about what you learn here, of the benefits of Exercise, Rest, Nutrition and Hydration will congratulate you on the wisdom to which you're leading your life. So perhaps, and unless you have any major issues, you should try to reinforce all the pillars of your wellness and only then see if you need the often prescribed opinion of your GP.

So why do we lose our libido? There are many reasons, but here are the main ones:

STRESS

Both men and women suffer the effects of stressful situations in a variety of different ways and most of the time we learn just to cope. But 'feeling sexy' usually isn't the state we find ourselves in when under stress. Stress can come from our work or a lack of self-esteem, taking on too much or not being busy enough and having too much time on our hands. It also has a significant effect on the perfectionist – if you are too hard on yourself, or you have the need to control everything in your environment.

Your thoughts, feelings and actions will all be affected by the level of stress your body carries, your ability to recognise the symptoms can help you manage them in different ways and will contribute to your overall health. For example; by learning how to handle intimacy and specifically physical intimacy in a healthy way helps. For both men and women, this is extremely important, as sex would help combat stress, using sex as a stress management technique can invigorate your relationship, at a physical, emotional and mental health level, this technique will also bring good mood into the equation which is definitely a plus. But unfortunately, men report two major problems – anxiety about performance and climaxing too early (also known as Premature Ejaculation) according to the American sociologist, Edward Laumann. Almost one in three men report premature ejaculation, while around one in five is worried about performance.

And the anxiety doesn't stop there. Many modern, loving, and conscientious husbands feel they have not truly 'performed' unless their partners climax during sex, too. And as Laumann's statistics show, only 26% of women report that they always experience orgasm during sex, compared with 75% of men*. No wonder people feel the pressure – and performing under pressure can also lead to a loss of libido.

But can men win? Absolutely; they just need to be more in tune with their partners and try not to rush it think of it as a tender loving project where the reward has no measure and the return is hugely satisfying.

MEDICAL ISSUES

Serious medical conditions such as cancer, depression, cardiovascular disease, hypertension and diabetes can affect the blood flow of the body including the genitals. If this happens, it can wreak havoc on the libido.

Too much alcohol is often to blame for increasing desire yet ruining the performance. Shakespeare talked about the effects of alcohol brilliantly in Macbeth ...

"Lechery, sir, it provokes, and unprovoked; it provokes the desire, but it takes away the performance; therefore, much drink may be said to be an equivocator with lechery: it makes him, and it mars him; it sets him on, and it takes him off; it persuades him, and disheartens him; makes him stand to, and not stand to; in conclusion, equivocates him in a sleep, and, giving him the lie, leaves him".

ERECTILE DYSFUNCTION

But don't confuse the inability to gain and maintain an erection with libido. Erectile dysfunction and impotence aren't the same things. But ED certainly increases with age. It's quite uncommon to young people, only 12% experience it by age 40, but by 60, it's 18%, and then there's a sharp rise from the age of 60 to up to 30% of men.

Vasodilators (medication which increase the blood flow by widening the blood vessels) such as Viagra, Cialis, Levitra are excellent provided there's sexual stimulation. It is not recommended just to take a pill and then lay on your back for an hour, waiting for something to happen. Take it, and an hour later, go and kiss and cuddle and do all the lovely physically intimate things that will lead to stimulation and turning you on.

Hydration can definitely help this issue. Please refer to our *Hydration Module* to learn more about the power of water.

MENOPAUSE
A decrease in physical Intimacy and Sexual Desire

As we grow older, our oestrogen levels start fluctuating and then drop. Leaving us feeling emotionally and physically a mess. The symptoms of menopause can be challenging, and we tend to focus on the wrong side of it. One of the fascinating rewards could be the freedom, which the menstrual cycle doesn't bring. We should look at the entire life event as a gift instead of losing yourself in a state of depression because you mistakenly feel that part of which made you a woman has disappeared with age.

Menopause is the perfect time to start enjoying yourself and sex is a significant part of it. Yes, there are some downsides to it, and this is not to say that they should be ignored, but if you focus so strongly on the downsides you won't be able to see the upsides to this.

So, oestrogen levels are down! Now, what?

Well, did you know that with a healthy balanced nutritional lifestyle you could actually *improve* your oestrogen levels? Metabolic

Typing Advice is a science that helps you find what is right for your body at a cellular level. To find out what your body needs regarding macronutrients to help bring balance into your body. Check our *Moving Intimacy Into the Fridge* seminar.

Hormonal changes will also bring with them changes in stress and will cause not only an emotional roller coaster but will also come in the form of physical pain.

Some of the things that will help relieve this kind of pain are; choosing the right lubricant for you, making time for foreplay – and I mean teasing one another the day before then start playing with each other at least 30 minutes before bed time – making time for foreplay will help you get wetter. Please also try to avoid cleaning your vagina with soap and chemicals as this prevents natural bacteria from forming and causes a chemical imbalance in the vagina. The vagina is, in fact, self-cleaning, so there is not too much need for the use of these washes.

One of my mottos is 'use it or lose it' don't deny yourself from sex just because you are not in a relationship. Find a sex buddy. There is absolutely nothing wrong with that. But if that is not your thing then buy yourself a good toy. And remember self-pleasure can be of great help if other forms of sex hurt too much – and this can always be a shared experience.

PERFORMANCE ANXIETY AND LOSS OF LIBIDO

Most men who have sexual issues in their later life report that there are some causative factors. The first is performance anxiety, and climaxing too soon. These psychological issues should be dealt with by introducing a balanced wellness lifestyle approach. However, if the symptoms persist and they are not 'normal' you should visit your doctor to discuss these further. There is lots of help available, so address the problem, remember that you're NOT alone, and get some help so you can stop suffering in silence.

For men, sexuality tends to be focused disproportionately on the genitals. Focusing on the other erogenous zones can ease performance pressure – and add new pleasure. Where sexual satisfaction is concerned, the shortest distance between two points – from arousal to orgasm – is not necessarily a straight line. Take detours along each other's body. Be 'pleasure oriented', rather than 'goal oriented'. Tease, touch and take your time but above all do it purposefully and without any expectations or pressures. As if has been said in other chapters, a massage shared between a couple is all about the intention behind the touch and the way we touch each other, rather than the massage itself.

Stress and loss of libido is an often-overlooked issue within sexuality and intimacy, especially when it comes to men. Two examples of clients will illustrate what I mean. In one case, a client came to me with a problem, which most men can only dream about, every man's fantasy, but it wasn't long before it proved to be a hindrance rather than a fantasy.

And in the other case, lack of attention to the body, allowing unnecessary ill health to intervene in a previously healthy lifestyle, which caused a series of difficulties with intimacy between the couple. The wife in this scenario was on anti-depressants that severely affected her libido, and he suffered from sleep Apnoea, so they resorted to having separate bedrooms.

To learn more about the importance of REST visit our 3-part blog
Start Getting Quality Sleep.

Let's talk about the first set of clients. Charles – not, of course, his real name – his wife, Claudia and Claudia's girlfriend Anne. Yes, you read that correctly. Charles' wife had a girlfriend and was quite happy to share her with him, but although it was something which initially he welcomed and enjoyed, it soon became a problem. But let me start at the beginning.

Charles and Claudia were married in the early 1980s and children soon came their way. Outwardly, they were the happiest of couples. He had a terrific job as a lawyer with loads of prospects, and he was well rewarded. She was a professional woman, also a lawyer, and had her own working society and earned good money. Claudia often travelled in her work as a lawyer and wined and dined clients. She was lucky enough to be often accompanied by Charles.

At home, their marital life was pleasant, but far from exciting. They made love once a week, usually on the same night, usually in the same way. But when she was in the midst of a difficult case, she would ask him to release her from the commitment of making love, citing exhaustion as an excuse.

As time went on, they no longer made love, though they held hands, cuddled, kissed and fondled each other.

Eventually, Charles confronted Claudia and asked her why she no longer wanted to have sex with him. At first, she used exhaustion as an excuse. But as he continued the cross-examination, she admitted that she no longer found sex with him appealing. He asked whether it was him, or if there was another reason. She told him that it was him and then, almost under her breath, she said that it was not just him, but any man.

Stunned, and being able to read a subtext when he heard it, he asked her whether she was more inclined towards women than men. At the beginning of their marriage, she didn't realise that she was bisexual. So she admitted she was, in fact, strongly inclined towards women but she did enjoy sex with him when she was in the mood. And then, having breached her walls of self-imposed secrecy, she told him that she was having an affair with another lawyer in the firm, a younger woman called Anne.

It had begun at an international conference. They were discussing difficult points in a presentation Claudia was making the following day, and as they became physically closer and closer, they'd kissed, fondled and gone to bed. It was Claudia's first lesbian experience, and she'd orgasmed stronger and more intensely than ever before.

Charles was stunned, mystified, hurt, offended, but he loved his wife and tried to be an understanding husband. He told Claudia that if she wanted to continue with this relationship, that it was all right with him, provided they maintained the closeness, warmth and love, which had been so much a part of their marriage.

And that's the way things remained for five years until Anne started to sleep over. They all went to bed together, and Claudia was particularly turned on when she watched Charles and Anne make love.

So why did they come and consult with me? Why did they need therapy when all of them … Charles, Claudia and Anne … were so sexually, physically and emotionally satisfied?

Because Charles wasn't emotionally satisfied. Sexually, he had everything he wanted in life, and who could blame him, a loving and attentive wife and a willing girlfriend whom they shared. It was every man's sexual fantasy; but for Charles, it wasn't intimate. Not by a long way. And what Charles desired more than anything was the emotional bond he had once enjoyed so very much with his wife. It was as if sharing her with Anne was a weakening of that bond. He hid it from the two women, and to some extent himself, but it eventually became overwhelming, and he had to deal with it through the intermediation of a professional counsellor. A lot of his insecurities emerged because of this, and Claudia was the first to recognise the problem. It was she who made the appointment to come and see me.

It had taken just three sessions before it became apparent that the insecurities originated with Charles' mother. He came from a large family of children; he was the third to be born, the first two being twins. And after him came a daughter who was born profoundly deaf.

Growing up Charles always had the impression that his childhood, and especially the love of his mother, was shared with others. And indeed, on closer questioning, it became obvious that she spent most of her emotional time with the other children and his deaf sister, all of whom had greater needs than that of Charles, who was independent, almost from the time he could walk. So the emotional bond that should have been the very foundation of his life wasn't as present or noticeable as it is with other children. Which meant that when he met and married Claudia, the bond that was so thin and vapid in his childhood could become strengthened and only matured into his adult life.

So when, after 16 years of marriage, the bond, which had been Charles' mainstay, was suddenly weakened and fractured, and subsequently overtaken by Claudia's extramarital affair, he felt bereft emasculated and diminished.

The story of his minimisation in the relationship (perhaps imposed by them or perhaps self-imposed) reached its climax when, after a full day in court, he met the women for drinks in a city centre hotel.

They suggested that they book a room, have room service, and have an orgiastic sexual romp. But Charles couldn't face reality, and paid for their room, their romp, their food and drink, and went home ... to an empty bed, a lonely bath and the sleep of a frustrated bachelor.

What to do? What did I advise? I asked him to see me privately, without his wife being there. I said that I thought the women, especially his wife, were being selfish. They had gone out and found satisfaction in themselves, and even though they included him, it was more by way of tolerance than acceptance. I told him to take Claudia out to dinner, and in a quiet and reflective conversation, I suggested that he should be allowed to confront his feelings. First to Claudia then to Anne.

Claudia accepted his desire, and so the three of them got together, and Charles told them that even though he was included, he felt that the very foundation of his life with Claudia was being fractured. He told them that he wanted an end to their affair and that he wanted Claudia back.

But things didn't work out well. After tears, recriminations and pain ... lots of pain ... Claudia made it clear to Charles that she wanted to remain with Anne. So they separated.

That's not the end of the story, however, Claudia and Anne didn't last long, and Claudia asked to return to Charles for 'another try'. He refused, and Claudia took up with another lover, this time a man. That affair lasted only four weeks.

Charles is alone, but dating women, and seeking a long-term relationship. Many young female barristers find him attractive, and he could easily bend one or more of them. But he doesn't want to. He wants to find one woman who will allow him to build the emotional as well as the physical intimacy, which, he so badly, desires.

His penis no longer has a brain of its own and now marches to the beat of his heart or at least his emotional state. This is when most men get confused and think that it is their age or body's declining, but this isn't necessarily so. Often, this is part of the reality of being human and having emotions. It also has nothing to do with the new partner as it does take time to build intimacy and especially physical intimacy.

Another case of lack of sexual intimacy happened at roughly the same time that I was trying to assist Charles; in this case, Phillip came to me along with his wife, Elizabeth. She was a long-term sufferer of depression and had been prescribed Prozac and other anti-depressants. And to compound the physical side of their marriage, he was suffering badly from sleep Apnoea and snoring like a buzz saw. So he was to sleep in another bedroom. This naturally causes massive problems for their sex lives. Tell me have you ever tried to have sex with your wife or partner while sleeping in the other room? They hadn't had sexual intimacy in months, probably much longer and along with the sexual intimacy; the emotional intimacy had left the house.

As a businessman, Phillip had to go overseas, and on one of the trips, he went to Jakarta, where, in a hotel bar he met an Indonesian woman called Sayarika. They had a passionate affair, and when he came back, he made the excuse that he had to return to Indonesia again within the next three weeks. It was, of course, a patent excuse and although he covered the situation as best he could, both of them knew that it was all a lie. He had a wonderful time in Indonesia ending up in a week-long stay on the island of Bali, where they did what young people do, even though Phillip was a balding middle-aged man, and Sayarika was a 30-something housewife.

Even though he was getting regular holidays in Indonesia, and playing like a schoolboy with his new toy, his relationship with Elizabeth seemed to deepen. And then a miraculous thing happened. The pressure of needing and wanting sexual intimacy was no longer there, and so a considerable amount of inner tension dissolved. He lost a significant amount of weight and his sleep Apnoea improved dramatically. They became close friends again, laughing and joking and discussing and holding hands, as they had when they were first married. Before the troubles had entered their relationship.

They didn't fall back into bed immediately, but they did regain quite a lot of their emotional intimacy. Soon, they desired more than closeness and comfort; they were once again sexual. Until suddenly and completely unexpectedly, Phillip got a phone call from Indonesia … from Sayarika. It was one of those conversations, which sent shivers down his spine. Sayarika told him that unless he told his wife about her, and leaves her, then she would tell her and that would be the end of their marriage. Phillip didn't believe her, and for a year, Sayarika continued to threaten, even though Phillip no longer saw her, and had stopped going to Indonesia. But a couple of months afterwards, living a close and sexual relationship with Elizabeth, his wife, received a phone call from Indonesia. A phone call which was a cry from an abandoned woman in Jakarta who felt as though she'd been overthrown.

Elizabeth refused to allow Phillip to leave to go overseas on business, and he was forced to sleep in another room. He told her that he needed sexual and physical intimacy and that he didn't want to lose her as a friend. He laid it on the line. He said that at the time, he needed sexual contact and intimacy. He mentioned time and time again that he had needs and that she wasn't available because of her worry about her depression and that he felt it was unfair for him to continue putting his own needs on hold, especially after so many years of waiting for her, and that at the same time he didn't know what to do and how to handle the situation. He also mentioned that for a long time he had not felt wanted as a man and that Sayarika was able to shine some light onto that place inside of him that he felt that Elizabeth had a responsibility to provide for his physical needs, just as he supplied all of her needs as a woman and a wife. Or at least come to a joint agreement without sacrificing so many years of marriage. They are still together growing other aspects of intimacy as they have purchased a country house that they are happily building together and are slowly but surely bringing their lives back under control and most importantly they are doing it together.

Happiness is not the absence of problems; it's the ability to deal with them in a healthy way! It is my belief that the source of unhappiness can be shifted but one thing rings true, and that is that the source of unhappiness always has been and always will be there. However what we do have the power to change is the perception of it, and accept the challenges, the key events, and all the situations that compose our human conditions and together, we should empower ourselves with as much understanding as possible to master the challenges in a better and more positive way.

CHAPTER FOUR

So ... What do food exercise and
rest have to do with all of this?

Well, EVERYTHING.

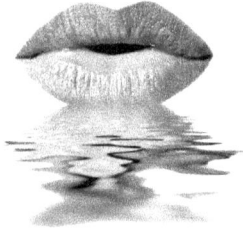

*You earn your body; sexercise is
an awesome way to get fit.*

In the previous chapter, we dealt with health problems and sexual activity. But while increasing age often leads to increasing health issues, most of us remain healthy or can be medicated to maintain a normal lifestyle. Unfortunately, the meaning of 'normal' somehow has been lost in translation as more often than not we choose the route of allopathic treatment rather than holistic. Allopathic is defined as 'treating the symptoms', which doesn't take into account what might be the underlying cause of the problem. It relies on drugs, which are often worse than the diseases that they are supposed to be treating. I am personally against reductionist medicine, and I strongly recommend you also use common sense when making decisions when it comes to your body.

So assuming that you can function in a normal adult way, assuming that you exercise regularly and sensibly, that you do care about the kinds of food you consume and that you have enough physical and mental activities to energise your mind. It is time to talk about nourishment, review your physical activity and check in with your body's natural rhythm. In other words, ways of improving your sex life.

Yes, Food, Exercise and Rest (notice the capital letters) are the three essential ingredients of an erotic, intimate sexual lifestyle.

You eat, you exercise, and then you rest, and it all directly relates to intimacy.

If you overeat, eat junk food, or fill your body with unhealthy foods, which provide instant gratification but no long-term residual nutritional benefits, then intimacy takes a downward spiral. If you are full of the wrong stuff, it's hard to get a hard-on or to want to receive a man's (or woman's) sexual approach if you feel bloated and uncomfortable or even worst constipated.

If you never exercise, sit at your desk for hours on end, or find even getting out of a chair to be the cause of twinges, aches or pains. Then hugging, kissing, and fondling doesn't feel the same as when you were young, and your body was attuned to eroticism.

Finally, if you don't rest, but spend hours every night watching television, or sitting over a long meal, or lounging in a chair drinking that tenth bottle of beer. By the time you want to be intimate, you'll find that your hormone level is at low ebb, and the desire might be there, but the performance won't be. The sad thing about this is that we hide behind the excuse that this is what life has to offer or even worse is that people often use obesity as a cover up.

So my question to you is, what is your obesity protecting you from? Obesity has become an epidemic and relationships are suffering because sex becomes exceptionally difficult for extremely overweight people. It isn't a joke it's a very real, frustrating and debilitating phenomenon.

It's an old but true cliché; 'we are what we eat'. Food, without any doubt, is our best medicine, or our worst enemy and is the only way our body will have the energy to perform at its best or suffer the consequences of its ill effects.

If our hair is too long, or our nails need touching up, we can go to a hairdresser or a manicurist; but if we've put on so much weight that we need new clothes, then, unfortunately, there's no hiding the fact. And often, spoken or even unspoken comments from friends or family can hurt us to the very depth of our souls. That's when we often replace some of our friends who make bad or hurtful remarks for another friend the fridge.

But, like so much in our lives, we can change our weight, and we can change the way in which our body reacts. Not by giving up food (and going on one of those crazy lettuce-leaf diets), but by eating the right food, for us. How do we determine what the right fuel is for our individual selves? It's called Metabolic Typing Advice, and that's something we won't talk about now, but here is where you'll find what you need to know about *Metabolic Typing Advice*.

And here's the excellent news. Did you know that by exercising, you can actually help stimulate your sex hormones? If you're overweight or bordering on obese your immune system is jeopardised, and your self-image, your ego and your willpower devolve. But the moment you begin to lose weight by changing your lifestyle with wellness as a goal, your ego takes a boost, your willpower becomes stronger and more challenged and the image you have of yourself (every time you look in a mirror, or somebody says to you that you've lost weight and are looking slimmer) goes through the roof.

And yes!!! This, in turn, affects your sex hormones, which are boosted by the prospect of renewed sexual activity coming back into your life.

We shouldn't go to the gym to lose weight. We may shed kilos, but this is a beneficial by-product; we should go to the gym or start an exercise routine to feel better, to get the endorphins charging around our bodies so that we feel terrific and regain our confidence. Men, who are overweight, tend to have less testosterone and more oestrogen in their bodies than men who are of normal weight. Studies have shown that in men who are over 40, each one-point increase in body mass index is associated with a two percent decrease in testosterone.

And Testosterone is the major male hormone that's responsible, among other things, for sperm production and libido. Obese men tend to have lower total and free testosterone levels as testosterone is converted to the female hormone in fat tissue and where there is too much fat the conversion is greater.

Here are some facts about the different categories of obesity:

Ideal (healthy) BMI is 18.5 to 24.9 kg of body fat
A BMI of 25-29.9 kg of body fat is overweight
A BMI of 30-34.9 kg of body fat is obese (Grade I)
A BMI of 35-39.9 kg of body fat is obese (Grade II)
A BMI of 40> kg of body fat is obese (Grade III) or morbidly obese

Have you got a tummy? Can you reach your penis when you go to the toilet? What do you think this does to your self-esteem? Are you hiding behind the hope that there is a magic tablet that will cure your obesity?

Is it a pure denial of reality that is leading your body to its present physical problem?

The trick is to find out why you are sabotaging yourself? If you believe that there is one correct way of eating, which applies to everyone, then you've probably fooled yourself into thinking that there is one form of diet which fits all. Your body processes food differently to everyone else, and so we should all eat the food, which is appropriate to our specific needs. Finding the right balance of protein, carbohydrates and fats to suit our individual bodies is the solution to this problem. Stop guessing what is right for you and start feeding your cells rather than your mind. And if you don't know the difference between protein, carbohydrates and fats, or you think that eating gluten free foods are the solution to your eating habits or that starvation is the shortest way to lose weight, then this is the wrong mindset, and you are in self-sabotage mode.

One of the biggest culprits is an evil, dangerous, nasty white powder sold for very little at you local supermarket. It's a legal product, yet it's abused by billions of people and leads to obesity, health problems and premature death.

It has a much bigger impact than cocaine does and on a much larger scale too.

I'm talking about sugar. Did you know that sugar hides behind 61 other names and that you probably are ingesting it right now without even knowing? These include familiar names such as sucrose and high-fructose corn syrup, as well as barley malt, dextrose, maltose and rice syrup, and the list goes on and on.

Don't get me wrong sugar is lovely with coffee and cake, but we have to restrict it, and possibly even lose it from our food intake as it is an addictive poison.

CASE STUDY NO. 1
You can't tell me obesity is OK!

One of my clients, a young woman, aged 27, who had an unsatisfactory sex and social life because she had been obese from the time she went to primary school, came to see me about her sexuality and sexual performance. She was advised to see me as she had discussed suicide with a friend of hers, who became seriously worried and begged her, to come to me.

Of course, it wasn't surprising that her parents were hugely overweight as well, and when she was little more than a baby, they thought that they were doing their daughter a favour by treating her with a regular supply of sugary sweets and chocolates.

The moment she arrived at her primary school, the headmistress called the parents and advised them that they should put her on a diet, but they assured the headmaster that all would come good in the end and that her life would be happy, even if she were a little bit overweight.

When she came to see me, she was anything but happy. Her sex life was a mess, and she was finding it increasingly difficult to manage a relationship well. She was sad, lonely, and thinking herself a failure even before she'd begun to set her feet correctly on the path of life. I knew that she had a problem with self-image, but one that could be cured with good advice (that her parents needed as well), empathy, and more than just a little bit of straight talking.

Soon she began opening up to me about her first boyfriend;

"I am tired of hearing people talking about how I should get over my body image and learn how to accept myself as I am, to be completely honest there is nothing sexy about being obese, especially when trying to have a healthy sex life. I used to be 149 kilos and had sex with someone who was probably 204 Kilos. So we had to negotiate sexual positions. It's kind of ... hard to do sometimes. It depends, though. Doggy style didn't work. My butt was too big, and his dick was too small. When we tried it, he would sort of pick up his stomach and put it on my back and then he would take his hands and pull my ass cheeks apart. Wow, that sounds gross when I come to think about it. And I didn't cum if you see what I mean.

"Missionary was probably the best thing, with some pillows under me. Even then it wasn't pleasurable because of our fat just getting in the way.

"He also broke his bed all the time. He had his bed frame on bricks and would still crack it or bend it. We broke the bed three times over our relationship, and there was at least one time when I was there that the bed made a horrible noise and sort of jolted. I'm sure something broke. We tried to ignore it but it was all I could think about for awhile, and that just distracted and made it harder to focus on us. I'm sure his dick would have been a lot bigger had he not been morbidly obese. But blow jobs and fingering were honestly much easier than full sex most of the time, so that's what happened".

She told me that while he was sexually satisfied, she wasn't and she was going mad. So I told her about different sexual positions she could try, and I also gave her the tools to start changing her lifestyle with good nutrition and a gentle exercise regimen which, I'm thrilled to say, began to work within a month and she began feeling a lot better for it. She has now lost a lot of weight, looks terrific, and is attracting men who are vastly more capable of having sex in a much less complex way; they have been able to satisfy her emotionally and physically. Some people in her position would have given up, but after our first session and once I had opened her eyes to all the possibilities that lay ahead for her future, she was determined to living a healthier sex life and so that is why she chose to lose the weight.

During our discussions, I had created a template of different positions for sexual activity for herself and her partner. I'd like to share them with you, so you know that there are ways you can enjoy an active sex life until you lose the weight to make it more fulfilling:

The Fine-tuned Missionary Position

If you're into vanilla sex, then here's a variation for people who are obese. The basic missionary position, which is the man on top of woman, can prove difficult when you're dealing with a large belly and if your partner has a large tummy, then it's even more challenging. But change the situation a little bit by fine-tuning the position ever so slightly, and you and your partner can still manage to enjoy the intimacy and ease of the most popular position. Rather than the man lying on top of the female, he can kneel or rest between her legs as he penetrates her. And while he's down there, he can use his tongue to good effect. Just one quick secret, when you're down there, don't move your head. Yes, you heard me DO NOT MOVE YOUR HEAD – you're not looking for something. Keep your head still, and use your tongue as if you were slowly remember … licking an ice cream! Oh and now that we are on the subject, it seems that some men do not enjoy going down on women, so perhaps you should honestly talk about this before you make the trip down under!

WOOF! WOOF! If You Get What I Mean …
Ok, for those who don't it's called Doggie Style

This has got to be one of the greatest sex positions for men and women who are overweight – While it may not give you the same intimacy that comes from a face-to-face position. I know that it is wonderful to look your partner in the eyes while you're making love, because we're all visual creatures, the idea of mounting, or being mounted from behind, is incredibly erotic. But if you're a woman, there's an additional benefit, because doggie style enables a man to stimulate the front wall of the vagina, which dramatically improves the chances of hitting the g-spot and allowing you to gain one of the strongest, teeth-clenching orgasms on the record books. And of course, entering a woman from behind enables her to use her fingers to rub, massage and pleasure her clitoris. If you're a man, encourage your partner to do so, even if they're a bit nervous about doing so, because it's akin to masturbation, with all the social prohibitions and taboos, which have been built up by the churches against pleasuring ourselves.

Spooning, Mooning and Swooning

Spooning … laying on your sides as he enters from behind is a superb way for pregnant, overweight and obese people to have sex. There's no weight involved by having one lay on top of the other. But penetration can be tricky because of the layers of fat, and so using a couple of pillows to prop up the hips to a more comfortable level is one way to gain the correct position to reach the satisfaction you crave. The man can also prop up her top leg as he pushes his penis into her vagina, and hold onto her body to increase penetration as he thrusts.

'Hey, I Want To Be On Top'

If the woman goes on top of the man, then the size of his penis becomes less of a problem. When she's on top she can position herself comfortably for penetration and control the depth and speed of the sex ... and isn't depth and speed what great sex is all about? The advantage for the man is that he then gets to lay back, enjoy the view and the feeling of his partner doing the hard work. This is one of the primary reasons that overweight men prefer this position. It's relaxed, and she does the grinding and grunting, and he's just there for the ride ... so to speak.

So there you have a few ideas to get you going while you are on your journey to self-improvement and a life of sexual satisfaction. One last thing sex should be fun and enjoyable and if it doesn't work sometimes – stay, play, touch, accept and forgive ... above all enjoy the time together.

Moving Towards Wellness

Let me introduce you to a chemical, which is floating around your body. Please meet this culprit of a friend! It's called Cortisol, and it is produced when your body is under both physical and or mental stress. Cortisol is released from the adrenal glands and is the beginning of the 'fight or flight' human response. When we were prehistoric tribal – Proto-Sapiens – walking around jungles and savannahs, we always had to be on the lookout for hungry lions or tigers. So it was cortisol, which was released the moment we heard a beast's roar, and we either ran like crazy to the nearest tree or froze and succumbed to the hunger of a lion.

But these days few of us are chased by lions or tigers, however, the constant stress we're under; traffic, sudden noises, frustrations, demands by bosses, sleeplessness, anxiety or perhaps the fear of our credit card being rejected in front of a snooty shop assistant, mean that cortisol is being released all the time. Sure in tiny amounts but it's now become public health enemy No.1.

Increased levels of cortisol have an adverse effect on learning and memory; it lowers our immune system and decreases our bone density. Causing us to gain weight, spiking an elevation in our blood pressure, increasing the bad cholesterol and causing heart disease. And that isn't the end of the problems, but you get the picture.

Elevated levels of cortisol also cause mental problems such as an increased risk of depression, mental illness and lowering your life expectancy.

So let's put one thing right out there, front and centre.

STRESS ISN'T A TROPHY! SO WHY DO WE CARRY IT WITH US EVERYWHERE WE GO?

It seems to me that we are all searching for inner peace, but as soon as life becomes too calm, we appear to go out of our way to seek excitement. Athletes are well known for this. They're adrenaline junkies, always looking for the next endorphin hit.

Many of us go in search for more and more cortisol and epinephrine hits. Why is it we are addicted to these adrenaline spikes produced by strong emotions such as fear or anger, which causes an increase in heart rate, muscle strength and blood pressure? All of which are factors contributing to metabolic syndrome, sometimes known as obesity, cardiovascular diseases and type 2 diabetes. These disorders in most cases are preventable by just adjusting to a better lifestyle.

So, how do we know when our bodies are out of balance?

a) If you have trouble sleeping or even when you have slept all night you feel tired in the morning.
b) If you are gaining unwanted weight despite eating right or exercising.
c) If you are prone to catching colds and or other infections easily.
d) Craving unhealthy food is yet another giveaway.
e) Not to mention that your sex drives are in the crapper.

f) You've noticed that your guts have been acting up.

g) Even feeling blue and anxious is another giveaway.

Most people will take themselves to the gym or put themselves in the hands of an inexperienced trainer and believe that any exercise is better than none!

So let's make something very clear, everything you do or don't do for that matter, will have an effect on your body thus the stress from excessive exercise would just be stacked onto whatever daily stress life throws at you. So the rule number one is to learn how you can achieve balance to avoid running out of power.

I strongly suggest you start with a 'prescribed exercise' program that will cater to your specific needs and levels of stress; this will be beneficial to you as movement and exercise are paramount to feeling better and help to decrease the release of cortisol and in improving your mind and body connection. But when beginning this training and exercise, I want you to be aware that when you went to your primary school, the teachers didn't instruct you in material given to university students, did they? I ask that you treat this new found routine, in the same way, being walking or join a gym. But no matter how good the others look in their lycra shorts and tight vests, remember that you're a primary school level exercise beginner. Just because they can bench-press 180 pounds, don't think that you can too, or you'll just end up doing yourself serious damage. And this is what so many personal trainers don't know or aren't trained in. They think that 'burn baby burn' is the way to get fit. But people like me; trained in C.H.E.K, tailor individual and proper food intake, exercise, hydration, relaxation and willpower regimens to our clients with their specific needs taken into consideration.

CASE STUDY NO. 2
Multiple orgasms …

Anybody would have called her a nymphomaniac, yet I didn't agree. Firstly, it is my role to be non-judgmental, and secondly, society judged her by its standards, which were not the same as hers.

My client, the lady in her mid-40s who came to see me because of the criticisms she was getting from her mother, her sister and her ex-husband, were driving her crazy and she was even beginning to doubt herself her sanity and her moral compass.

Her name is Annette. And of course, to protect her identity, this is not her real name. So Annette came to me and said, 'I think I'm a nymphomaniac, and I need treatment.'

Once we had spoken at great length about her sex life, it was evident to me that she wasn't a nymphomaniac, but somebody who had a healthy, beautiful, open and varied relationship with her body, and the men ... and women ... and toys she invited to join her.

Annette is an accountant and spends much of her day consulting to clients in their offices. She's tall, strikingly attractive (the very definition of a MILF) which has meant that she has always received admiring glances from clients of the firm and their employees.

Not that she played to the gallery, but she did wear clothes, which were more appropriate to a 30-year-old than a woman in her mid-40s. White blouses, often opened to the swell of her breasts, a skimpy bra, which would just show through her blouse, skirts which ended just above her knees, black stockings, high heel shoes, and often a choker of jet black leather around her neck which many of the men in the offices would have seen in porn.

So while it was never her intention, her very appearance in an office shouted, 'Hey boys, look at me.'

But to her, looking like that was a sign that she was a woman doing a professional job looking her best. Many of the men, and some women, in the offices she visited, didn't view her in that light. Rather, they saw her as a target for their sexual desires.

After all looking her best was sexy, attractive and very chic.

And it wasn't all one way. She was strongly attracted to many of the men she met and being a divorcee she was ready, willing and able. The only thing that held her back was her professional ethics of screwing with a client or his employees.

Up until the time that she went to see a new client, a mid-sized Advertising agency where the men wore open shirts and sneakers – ties and jackets were banned – and the women looked as if they were at Saturday morning coffee.

It had taken her two visits before she found herself in a locked door toilet for the disabled, a very convenient and accessible bathroom on the ground floor, having sex with one of the very attractive partners.

She arranged to meet him two days later, and to her considerable surprise when she entered his apartment she found his secretary in the kitchen making cocktails and wearing ... well ... not much more than an apron.

Annette had had experience with women when she was at University, and the threesome was one of the most exciting experiences she'd had sexually in many years. And she came. Strongly. Many, many times. She lost count because as she went from her to him to her and back to him, and he entered her and her and her, her orgasms seemed to blend one into the other until she tried to stand to go to the loo and found that she nearly collapsed on the floor. But she knew that she could handle it and afterwards, went back into the bed-arena, and repeated the main course again and again.

Of course, though Annette was considerably older than the man's secretary and older even than the man himself she was a regular at the gym, exercised at home, went for power walks every morning, and ate a healthy diet.

The party, which Annette had enjoyed was sometimes repeated and sometimes the man brought women other than his secretary into the bed.

But after six months Annette wanted other sexual experiences, and so she went with a girlfriend to a swinger's club in the city where she lived. There, with due sexual protection, as she watched a pole dancer do her thing she noticed that a man and a woman has been eyeing her for quite some time. He led her to a room full of mattresses where men and females were laying and making love. The man laid her down while the other woman undressed her and proceeded to have intimate sexual contact with her.

While she was in the middle of her fantasies, she realised that the man had lain beside her and was about to enter her. Again, she orgasmed and orgasmed until she was dry-throated and barely able to walk.

A month later in another client's office, she found that one of the employees was coming on strong. Remembering her encounters in the swinger's club, and suddenly sexually excited, she agreed to meet him for drinks, which inevitably led to bed.

And so her life continued with numerous sexual encounters with men and women in all different places.

Until her mother, a lady in her early 70s realised that her daughter was 'up to no good' as she told her. Her mother brought her sister into the conversation and then Annette's ex-husband, for some reason, and the pressure and accusations that she was a whore and a slut and a nymphomaniac hit her so hard she couldn't handle the pressure.

When she'd finished her story I said to her that to me; she was a totally normal, sexually adventurous woman who was harming nobody and glorying in her sexual satisfaction.

I asked what she wanted people to think about her, with no preconceptions of what was and wasn't moral behaviour.

She said that she wanted to be accepted, but that she was enjoying the sex so much. So why, she asked me, should she alter her behaviour? She said that when she was 90, she wanted to look back on her life, and say to herself that she had experienced what she had wanted to experience and that her life had been lived to the fullest extent possible.

I nodded and told her that she had two alternatives. One was that she could lead life according to other peoples' expectations, behaving as they considered to be a good daughter/sister/friend, regardless of the effect it had on her psyche. The other alternative was to go on living the life she was living provided she wasn't using, hurting or harming anybody; and that the way in which her mother and sister and especially her ex- viewed her was their problem, not hers. If they couldn't accept the woman that she was then, they had to change or get out of her life.

She thought about what I was saying, and then asked, 'But what if I became a prostitute? What if I charged men and women for the sex I currently give for free? Would my mother and sister have a right to criticise me?'

I told her that yes, they would be entitled to, but prostitutes who gave their bodies for money weren't hurting anybody. It was an old, famous and perfectly valid profession, which had been demonised by the Christian churches for 2016 years. And it seems to me that we judge the job based on what we know about prostitution from pop culture – crime movies and TV shows, all or most which portray the illegal, back-alley trade. Girls dominated by pimps and crippling addictions to illegal substances climbing into cars with total strangers and placing themselves at risk.

Yes, she could become a prostitute if she wanted to and if her mother and sister objected then it was their issue to deal with.

And then we got back to the enviable situation of her multiple orgasms. Was it wrong for a woman to have so many? To have them one after the other, whereas most women don't orgasm at all, or if they are lucky, enough they may just have one.

I explained that she was a healthy woman who exercised regularly and ate properly, someone who felt good about her sexuality and herself. And that, I explained, was her good fortune.

Then I went on to tell her about Dr. Edward Group, who published an article where he said, 'There is no debate, regular exercise is vital for maintaining health and wellness.' Again and again, research confirms that everyone can benefit from physical activity. Want to live a long, healthy life? Your chances of doing so are far better if you regularly work your body.

I told her that research had found that exercise helps to shed inhibitions and that women sometimes orgasmed while exercising.

Dr. Group went into detail listing the most influential side effects of exercising:

a) Improve chronic fatigue syndrome symptoms
b) Puts insomnia to bed
c) Supports healthy pregnancy
d) Softens ageing
e) Improves mental health
f) Fights antidepressants

LIBIDO AND DEPRESSION

The University of Texas at Austin conducted a study involving 47 women who reported a decline in sexual arousal caused by antidepressants. Researchers had the women watch three erotic film clips during which time they measured genital arousal. Before two of the sessions, the women exercised. The results? Exercising before exposure of arousal inducing material increased genital arousal and sexual satisfaction.

The point I am trying to make is that and if this doesn't give you reason enough to start you exercising I really don't know what will.

Italian researchers put a small group of obese women with sexual complaints in a supervised weight-loss program (that included diet and about 10 hours of low-intensity exercise per week), they not only lost an average of 15 kilos but also reported higher levels of vaginal lubrication and the sexual frequency with a partner after 16 weeks. The study authors said, that weight loss does more than improve body image: It also helps improve insulin resistance. Overweight women whose bodies can't use the hormone to process glucose also tend to have lower levels of testosterone, which dampens self-confidence and sexual response.

LACK OF REST

If you want to know what one of the most successful killers of intimacy between partners is you need to look no further than the failure of providing the body with plenty of rest.

This happens due to stress, overeating, over-drinking, being overweight and snoring – some of the sleep disorders we seriously need to become aware of are:

- Continuous Positive Airway Pressure (CPAP)
- Delayed Sleep Syndrome
- Drowsy Driving
- Insomnia
- Narcolepsy
- Restless Legs

- PLMS was often known as Sleep Apnoea whether it'd be Obstructive or Central
- Shift work and the list go on …

We all lead busy lives, and so many of us make the excuse that we have to get things done and that's often a big mistake. Without a doubt sleep deprivation can lead to serious health problems, so please do yourself and your relationships a favour and don't trade your precious sleep hours for work hours.

Before the Industrial Revolution, people woke with the sun and went to bed with the rising of the moon. Then the artificial light was made universal through gas and electricity; factories were able to work through the night and sleep patterns changed. In the old days, the recipe for a balanced life was eight hours of sleep, eight hours of play and eight hours of work. Today, people are often lucky to get five or more continuous hours of uninterrupted sleep, and very little rest in between. So although we might not realise it, we are often at the lower end of the scale when it comes to physical, mental 'rest and relaxation'. Sleep deprivation can have serious consequences for health and welfare. No, I'm not talking about an occasional sleepless night, but times in our lives when we go for long periods without properly enabling our minds, brains and bodies to shut off. And that's when our bodies repair themselves and our sleeping minds get rid of all the clutter that's built up during the day.

A new study published in the Journal of Sexual Medicine in March last year went to prove the power of sleep further, finding that a decent night's rest greatly enhances a woman's sex drive. They also found that lack of sleep lowers the level of testosterone thereby killing libido. Testosterone plays a vital role in a person's sex drive (especially in men) which is why not getting enough sleep can have a profoundly adverse effect on anyone's libido.

A chronically exhausted body has no room for intimacy, so how can you expect a healthy sexual and intimate relationship? When we are deprived of sleep and relaxation, there's no place in our minds, hearts and spirits for cuddles, kind words, love making, intimacy and sex. Sure, we might do it mechanically, but we know our hearts aren't in it. And often at this stage, when the sex is automatic, impersonal and unexciting, we seek explanations and excuses; we look for alternatives; other partners or the excitement of the chase after someone new. This can be a very dangerous time in a relationship especially if the foundations aren't solid.

Sometimes a holiday together can do wonders. Sometimes changing the current pattern of your lifestyle can assist, it can even be something small and seemingly trivial like putting on a favourite movie and insisting that you and your partner watch it together, with no distractions, rather than one of you disappearing into a study or being on your phone or checking emails.

Sleep plays a crucial role in your Physical Health, especially in your brain function. We all know that we feel great after waking up after a good and restful night's sleep. But recent research is showing us just how vital this sleep is. The evidence is now showing that sleep affects the body in ways which were never imagined, even five or ten years ago.

Scientists today understand how a lack of sleep affects such ailments as cancer (According to Dr. Gladden, cancer is not a reductionist phenomenon; cancer is a 'holistic phenomenon') and so it needs to be treated as such. People who aren't aware of the term 'reductionist phenomenon' can be assisted by a great analogy:

'A car is a very complex thing, but you can break it down to its individual parts and understand them in detail. We can know how these parts fit together and how they function when they are assembled. By understanding its parts and how they function together we can know absolutely everything important there is to know about a car'.

This is reductionism at its finest. Most of the sciences see things in this fashion because frankly, it works. By understanding all the little pieces and seeing how they fit together, you can understand the mechanisms. And understanding mechanisms gives you power over the process and ability to adapt it to many uses.

Can anger be broken down into its pieces? What pieces? The movement of the face is not anger; the reaction of the body is not anger; they are processes associated with violence, but they are not the things itself. Does understanding how the body functions when a person is angry help you understand anger? No, not in the slightest. Anger and all emotions for that matter can only be understood as a whole. You cannot put pieces together and get anger from them because the pieces do not convey the essence of anger. No one doubts that machine bolts, camshafts and pistons can convey the essence of a car. According to an article, I read by The Weiler Psi. Their function in creating and running a car is obvious. But there is no way to see the reactions of the body and understand how they can convey anger. The only way to read the responses of the body is to first understand the anger. Some emotions don't even elicit body reactions.

Can you apply any reductionism to this emotion? Take sarcasm. It is very clear when it is being conveyed, but there is absolutely no way to reduce this to a set of physical reactions. Sarcasm is neither the slow clap nor the look in the eyes, nor those two things combined because this emotion can be conveyed with different gestures. If you didn't know what sarcasm was, it would be very hard even to explain it. For that matter, the anger shown above would also be hard to tell. Why is that? Emotions are acts of consciousness and awareness is hard to explain because our minds and vocabulary is inherently reductionist and consciousness is irreducible. That is the problem in its most basic form.

You cannot approach consciousness with a reductionist mindset or with reductionist tools because none of this works in comprehending what consciousness is. Nowhere is this more evident than neurobiology? Reductionism has been highly successful in so many areas that one of the most fundamental problems with this approach has been virtually ignored.

Disease, obesity, depression and mood swings. There are more and more illnesses, which are now being exacerbated by the lack of sleep. It's alarming how many new illnesses are being worsened by this lack of sleep. In the past 30 years, smoking has been seen as the No. 1 cause of serious illnesses in the community. But sleep deprivation is fast catching up.

CASE STUDY NO. 3
A *separate bedroom* …

Recently, a middle-aged man and woman came to see me because of his lack of libido and her increasing frustration. Let's call him Oscar and her Lucy.

They'd been married, happily, for thirty years. At the beginning of their marriage, they had sex regularly, almost every night during the week, and a couple of times a day on weekends. And Lucy was always in hysterics with Oscar's stories and jokes. She often told him that he should have been a stand-up comedian.

Then the kids came along, and sex was still regular but stolen when the children were sharing their bed.

Then Oscar's career took off with a couple of excellent deals he had pulled off and so naturally, he was promoted. Ten years after they were married, he was offered a position on the Board of his company, which required a lot more work and frequent travelling to interstate and overseas affiliates.

To any outside observer, they were living a perfect lifestyle. They had a lovely house in a safe suburb; their kids were happy and well adjusted and did well in their schools. Lucy was involved in local politics and managed her own small local business.

As the kids grew, the sex was still regular, but vastly less adventurous, and they appeared to all intents and purposes to be living a life, which would be comfortable but vanilla.

But Lucy wasn't happy. She felt abandoned and deprived. She felt that while Oscar still loved her, his interests were elsewhere. Soon, she began wondering if his interests involved other women. Was that the reason that they only had sex once a week, and when they did, it was functional, unemotional and perfunctory?

He begged her to believe that there was nobody else in his life, but that he was so pressured at work, that he just didn't have the time or resources to split himself into a husband, lover, father and businessman.

When he put on weight over a two-year period, he began snoring, this ended in Lucy suggesting he sleep in the guest bedroom because he was depriving her of sleep. She had tried earplugs, to no avail, so the last resort was a separate bedroom.

This certainly had a devastating effect on their marriage. She knew that when she went to her room, he stayed up in his study and went to bed much later. She assumed that he was masturbating to porn when one day he was at work, she went into his computer and yet found nothing in his history which indicated he was viewing naughty websites.

So the only reason she could think of was that he was having an affair, and had lost interest. She confronted him, but despite his vigorous denials, she didn't believe him. Lucy contemplated hiring a private detective and discussed this with a close friend. Her friend asked her a simple question.

"Say you find out that he's having an affair. You'll divorce him? Right? And then what? Separate lives, destroyed family, divorce settlements, loneliness? Don't go in that direction, Lucy, go and see a wellness practitioner. See if there's an underlying cause to your problem. Don't give up on this".

Her friend told her that she'd been to one of my workshops, and when she understood the importance of balance in a person's life, she realised that this was precisely the sort of information Lucy and Oscar needed.

Fortunately, Lucy followed her friend's advice and came to see me. I listened to them both, and the depth of love between them was soon apparent, though it had been subsumed by layers and layers of complexity caused by careers, kids and much more.

So I began to ask Oscar a couple of questions, and his answers were incredibly revealing. I asked him whether his once-outrageous sense of humour had been lost? He said no; Lucy emphatically said yes! He was once funny; now, according to Lucy, he had lost the essence of his charm.

Was he, I asked, eating junk food? Oscar said that he wasn't bringing, but then admitted that he usually had a hamburger and chips when he was at work, because he was so pressured that he didn't have time for a proper lunch or fruit, salad and a sandwich.

Then I asked him if he had become more and more pessimistic. He said that he was the eternal optimist, but Lucy was emphatic that over the years, he had become increasingly negative. At the beginning of their marriage, he was the one who was adventurous and said that they should try new things and gain new experiences all the while, leading her increasingly to higher and higher levels of excitement. But over the past years, he'd become staid and boring and didn't want to do new things with her in case it led to failure.

I then asked if he was still affectionate. He said that he always kissed his wife, Lucy. She agreed but told me that his kisses were invariably just pecks on the cheek. The long loving kisses and cuddles were a thing of the past. I asked when he'd last bought Lucy a gift for a surprise, even as simple as a bunch of flowers. He laughed and said that they'd been married for 35 years, and these things didn't happen between long-term married people. Lucy looked stone-faced. And that told me a lot.

I'd quickly found what I considered the reason for their problem but wanted to ask a couple more questions to follow up. I asked Oscar how his self-esteem was. How did he appreciate himself?

He said that he was on his way to being offered the Executive Directorship of his company, and that made him feel great. But when I asked him how confident he felt in his abilities to do the job, another Oscar emerged.

One which was full of self-doubts that he could do what would be asked of him. And Lucy then chimed in and said that he was increasingly telling her that he didn't feel confident anymore in the way he was leading his life.

A couple more questions convinced me that sleep deprivation was the cause of most of their problems. I asked if he thought people considered him unattractive; I asked if he remembered the names and faces of people he should know, and he admitted that this was a problem, but he attributed it to being massively overworked. And so I told them that their problem was Oscar's lack of rest, lack of sleep, and perhaps sleep Apnoea (which I asked him to get checked by his GP for that). It was at this point that Lucy admitted that they weren't sleeping in the same room, due to his snoring.

Oscar told me that he slept perfectly well, and said that their problems weren't lacking rest or sleep, but must be due to another cause.

So I suggested that he and Lucy try something for a month. I told him to tell his colleagues that he wasn't able to read reports at night but would do them in the morning. I told him to cancel unimportant meetings called by other people, but only do meetings, which he called and considered necessary.

I told them to relax at night when he came home, and watch movies and start spending time with the kids and his wife. I told them to do twenty minute walks every night, and to count the hours they slept, to ensure that they both, yes both, slept seven hours a night.

I advised them to begin doing stretching exercises and to go to bed together at the same time every night. And I put them both on a special healthier food intake, a new lifestyle approach to ensure that they weren't overfilled in the evening and to cut out the regular glass of wine they had with dinner every night. Also no caffeine or stimulants after 5.00pm.

Why both? Why did I tell Lucy to do the same as Oscar? Because doing it on his own would have been isolating doing it in company with Lucy meant that it was a shared experience, they would remain accountable, and it would be more enjoyable.

They came back to see me a month later. Their lives were vastly improved.

Even in the first week of the new lifestyle, their relationship had improved, the power of their intimacy, which was once in crisis, was back to a true love affair.

It was remarkable. Oscar was sleeping better and more restfully, during the month they'd moved back into the same bedroom and their physical intimacy took on new and more adventurous pathways.

And it was all down to Oscar's lack of rest and sleep and high stress levels.

CHAPTER FIVE

The Good, the Bad and the Ugly ...

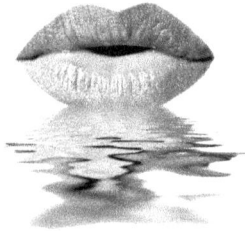

"There are a number of mechanical devices which increase sexual arousal, particularly in women. Chief among these is the Mercedes-Benz 380SL convertible."

P. J. O'Rourke

Pornography! Nasty, cheap, dirty, disgusting ... should be banned. Right? Wrong! Oh, so wrong.

Ok, some porn, especially that which tends towards violence and the degradation of adults, children and animals even is horrible.

But good, honest, clean (yes, clean!) and sexy pornography is just terrific and most certainly has it's placed in our lives. You read that correctly ... porn has a place in the often secret, hidden and guilty lives of 95% of the population.

One of the reasons we feel guilty watching pornography is because the Western Churches have determined that marriage has to be monogamous. The 39th President of the United States, Jimmy Carter, admitted to committing adultery in his mind, not his body when he said that at times he had lusted after a woman. That's the level of absurdity, which the churches have driven us to.

So, is monogamy a natural state of human life?

Well, I don't believe it is, no. Very few mammals in the animal kingdom have a one-on-one relationship, which lasts beyond reproduction. Women have traditionally sought one mate for child production, yes, but to stay with the same man throughout life is seriously limiting to our needs and our desires. It puts an inordinate amount of unnecessary stress and strains on our sexuality.

Women often desire what is forbidden to them by the strictures of Western culture. One of my clients admitted to me that though she was in a stable marriage, she had an overwhelming desire to be paid for sex.

"I don't want to become a prostitute. It is just a fantasy of mine to receive payment for sexual services, and it would be such a turn on if my husband actually paid me to perform these naughty things to please him every now and again. I want to pretend to be one of those girls we see in the XXX movies we watch together; they seem so sexually free and in control of their erotic power ... I want to feel what it's like to be in their shoes.

"I just find the idea of it so erotic, just the thought of knowing that I am explicitly doing such a dirty, erotic and often shamefully regarded thing, yet doing them with my husband in such a genuine and committed relationship is something that I find so enticing. The thought of such danger and yet feeling safe and secure is a fantasy that I have been considering talking to my husband Rick about to see if he would be up for a little role play".

As a Sex and Wellness Coach I need to let every single one of my clients explore their fantasies, yet be sure that they wholeheartedly understand that taking them into the bedroom and enacting such desires will, in practice, have a very different outcome and effect on their bodies – this does not necessarily mean it will be better or worse than they envision, it is just that it is going to be different and as long as they are ready to embrace the reality of the fantasy, whatever the outcome may be, then it is entirely up to them to take control over where they want to take their imagination.

So let me tell you the story of a monogamous couple who came to consult with me, Mia have been following my *enigma7 Wellness Program* for some time now, and so she was very familiar with me, this time she came to see me ask me a tough question. "Can I bring my husband in to discuss a very taboo subject with you?" She asked, and so we booked an appointment. They came together. And they had a story, which literally, blew me away.

Mia, a tall, beautiful woman in her young middle age, the sort of woman which young men refer to as a MILF ... a mother I'd like to f**k. She was sophisticated and sexy, but she had a problem, which she needed to discuss, and couldn't with her husband.

She had an overwhelming desire to be paid to have sex with a stranger. Yes, this gorgeous woman wanted to experience prostitution. Well, more like the feeling of liberation and control of what these women seem to have when it comes to freedom in the bedroom and pure eroticism; minus the inhibitions that were ruled by a doctrinaire family upbringing.

Ok, so that's a fantasy of many women, but few, and especially few like Mia, would ever take the plunge and tell somebody. It's a deeply hidden fantasy of far more women than men would ever realise. It was the transaction she wanted to experience, being paid to have sex, how it felt to be given money to lay with a stranger. No, she wouldn't enjoy the sex part, or indeed the intimacy, which was forced upon prostitutes, but a rather transactional side. Knowing that a man would pay good money to sleep with her, was her fantasy. When we fantasise, we don't tend to think about the bad side of sex, like the awfulness of a woman – or man – having sex with somebody they've never met before. But it's almost as if we want to touch the very core of our being, in our fragility, that we want to go against society's norms and acceptance. Call her a nonconformist if you wish. To be daring and naughty and breach the taboos which held society together.

So she told me what she wanted to do, and I explained how common this fantasy was. And then I asked her why she was telling me this. She said, "Because I want my husband, Rick, to know and I just don't know how I can bring it up with him, so he understands. I can't put it into words, without fearing his contempt, his condemnation. I need you to tell me how I can explain to him that I have this extraordinary fantasy".

I told her again that the only thing, which was astonishing, was that she'd told me what she wanted to do. And then I said, "Find a reason for inviting your husband to our next session. Tell him that you're here for counselling, and that I'd like to meet him".

Which she did. The following week, I met Rick. He was middle-aged, quite good looking, and obviously in love with, and caring of Mia.

We sat and talked and joked, and then, out of the blue, I asked him, "Tell me, Rick, do you ever watch pornography? How do you feel about it?"

He was shocked at first and looked at Mia for encouragement, but she smiled and nodded and said, "Well? Tell her".

So he did. He said that he watched it from time to time, especially when Mia was away from home on a business trip, but it wasn't something, which dominated his life and certainly not his relationship with Mia.

The session continued, and then there was another meeting and one after that, at which we skirted around the central issue. You can't just dive into the deep end until you've learned to swim.

So when I thought that the two were ready, I posed a question to Mia. I asked, "And tell me, Mia, what's your most intimate fantasy – say you weren't married, or in love with Rick – what would you most like to experience sexually?"

And she told him. He tried not to look shocked, but it didn't last because you could see from his eyes and his body language that he was so far removed from his comfort zone, that he wasn't sure whether to stand or sit, laugh or cry, congratulate her or condemn her.

I waited with bated breath until he spoke. She knew she'd probably gone too far, and excused herself, distressed, and walked out leaving Rick and me together.

He was distressed. "Oh God, I should have told her I'm fine with it. I'm stunned that she hasn't told me this before. We've been married 14 years, and this is the first time I've heard this. If she'd said years ago, I'd have arranged it for her.

"I'm a lawyer to a man who owns … well; let's call them houses of pleasure. One of them is an upmarket brothel in the best part of town. It would be such a pleased to be able to call him so that I can arrange it for us".

But I told him that he'd have to be careful of the way he did it. If it were obvious that he'd arranged it, then she'd feel guilty. There had to be a game, in which she had to win, but not know that he was on the sidelines, organising it all along.

It was only later that I found out, and realised how intelligent Rick was, and how attentive and loving of his wife.

One day, Mia was at home, doing some cooking for a dinner party she was organising that night. While the meat was in the oven, she opened her email browser and read her latest emails. And one of them bemused her. It was a woman she'd not seen since her college days. She greeted her and suggested that they meet in town for cocktails.

A delight to be reacquainting, Mia went a week later and waited at a table in the bar for her friend. Suddenly, without introduction, a man came and sat at her table. He apologised for disturbing her, introduced himself as Luke, and told her that he was a friend of the woman who'd written to Mia. He said that she was unwell, and had sent him in her place, just so that Mia wouldn't feel lonely.

They chatted, and within a half of an hour, Luke said,

"Look, I know you're married. So am I. How would you feel if we met again. I'm sure you'll say no, but if I don't ask, I'll never know".

Somewhat surprised, Mia said, "I don't think so. I'm very happily married, and I don't play around".

She was about to stand and leave, already planning what she'd say to her university friend when Luke said, "If I sweetened it? What would you say?"

"Excuse me? Sweetened it?" He nodded, and said, "Sure. How much to meet me again. Just for drinks?" Mia said, "You'd pay to meet me for drinks?"

"Sure would. You're a beautiful sexy lady. I'd love to pay for your time".

He handed over his business card, stood, and said, "Think about it. Call me if you're interested." And then he left.

She was stunned. She sat there for an hour in a state of shock. On the one hand, she was tingling with the excitement of what he'd said to her. On the other, she was horrified that he'd treat her like this.

A week later, she found his card in her wallet. A week after that, she plucked up the courage to phone him. Every hormone in her body was on supercharging when she heard him pick up the phone. "Hi, Luke, I don't know whether you remember me, but …"

"Hi Mia, I was hoping that you'd call. How are you? So, you've decided to meet me?"

They arranged to meet. And they did. And she had a splendid time, drinking cocktails in a bar. She'd dressed to kill, high heels, sheer black stockings, a little black dress, which clung to every part of her body, and her cleavage showed just sufficiently to be tantalising.

And at the end of the evening, as he kissed her goodnight at the entry to the cocktail bar before he put her into a taxi, he handed her an envelope. "Thanks for a wonderful evening. I hope you'll call me again".

She did. Because when the taxi pulled away, she found four crisp $50 notes.

But it took her a week to phone him. He recognised her voice immediately.

He asked her if she'd go to this address, and meet him there.

Four nights later, she stood outside the address he'd given her. It was a four, storey brownstone in one of the better districts of the city. She gathered up her spirits, not knowing what she was getting herself into, and knocked on the door.

An older, perhaps in her late sixties but very attractive lady answered, and said, "Come in Mia, you're expected".

She led her in. The house was beautifully furnished, with high-class tables and chairs, lounges, and chandeliers.

The woman, who didn't introduce herself, said, "I want to take your handbag. Leave it down here. And don't worry; it'll be perfectly safe. Now, there are a lot of lovely clothes for you to dress in. When the time is right, come back downstairs and chose something you like and get dressed in it. Meanwhile, follow me upstairs".

Too stunned to speak, Mia did what she was asked. She followed the lady upstairs, and out onto a balcony, where a vast and expensive table had been laid with cold meats, Champagne, tapas, nuts, canapés, and a variety of exotic fruits. It was like a buffet in an expensive hotel. She picked up a plate and helped herself to some of the food.

At this point, Mia was in total awe. She couldn't think and had lost all power to make any coherent decision. She was following the dictates of the moment, the place, and her desire to immerse herself in anticipation of what events were possible to happen next. But most importantly, she knew that she was totally safe.

After five minutes, Luke walked into the room, and then out onto the balcony. He kissed her on both cheeks and thanked her for coming. He was utterly calm. She was totally relaxed, yet she had no idea what he was thinking. Rick sprang to her mind. He poured her a glass of Champagne, and then he lit up a large cigar. Mia hated cigarettes and especially the stink of cigars, but somehow, on this one occasion, it added to the potential for naughtiness, to the magic in which she was immersing herself.

They talked for a few minutes. Mia wanted to ask him what was going on, but she knew that the wrong question could prick the bubble of the mystery, and so she continued with the light-hearted banter.

As if on cue, she heard the downstairs doorbell sound. A moment later, a beautiful, tall, elegant young woman walked into the lounge, and out onto the balcony. She apologised for being late, to which Luke responded, "You'll pay for it later. But for now, come and meet Mia".

They kissed, and she went over to kiss Luke. But unlike the cheek kiss for Mia, this young woman kissed Luke deeply on his lips, and Mia could see their tongues touching.

Luke then offered Mia a cigarette, which she refused. But the girl, who introduced herself as Sophie, lit one up, and the trivial banter continued, until Luke said, "Ok, it's time".

Then Sophie grabbed Mia by the hand, and led her through the lounge room, down the stairs, and into the room where all the clothes were.

"Chose what you want to be" Sophie said. Mia was desperate to ask her what would happen next, but that was part of the mystique for her. So instead, she merely went over to the racks and chose a lovely backless black dress. Sophie looked at it, and said, "That'll look hot on you".

Mia began to undress, but couldn't resist looking at Sophie as the beautiful busty girl quickly stripped off her dress, and exposed her firm breasts, her soft, pure white skin, and her shaved pubic area. She stood there completely naked, picked up a pair of crotchless panties, and pulled them on, followed by a corset and jaw-dropping demi bra.

"Is that all you're wearing?" Mia asked.

Sophie nodded. She came over and threw her arms around Mia.

"I'm told that this is your first time. Don't worry, it's wonderful, especially with Luke. He's very potent, hard as a rock. And if you don't want to, just say so, and he'll leave you alone".

The two women went back upstairs, and Luke was sitting in the lounge-room, waiting. She knew that everything was at his command. He stood, kissed both women, and led them into a nearby playroom, where he opened a suitcase and revealed all of the toys he was going to use. Diamond-decorated dog collars, black leather whips, stunning handcuffs, paddles, riding crops, Tantus pelts that looked like made of silicone, and much more.

Then he asked Mia to kiss Sophie's lips, and for her to play with Mia's ponytail, and they played together until he was visibly hard. Erect and expectant, he pulled Sophie to the couch, and he asked both women to undress him, while they were playing with each other. Then Luke pulled Sophie's leash and put her hands on the arms of the couch. He asked her to choose what instrument she wanted him to play with. He stroked the whip on her back, and she said, "No" so he tried a riding crop, and then a paddle until she agreed. Then he hit her softly, and she moaned. Then a bit harder until she was obviously in the pain of pleasure.

Mia was concerned. She'd never been in this position before. She didn't know what she was expecting, or whether she'd be willing to stay.

But then Luke told Mia to lay on her back, put her head in between Sophie's legs, and to lick her pussy ... Mia hesitated, as she knew she didn't like doing that, and yet she found herself obeying Luke's commands. Each time he'd stroke, Sophie, her body reacted and it made her push her pelvis forward forcing Mia to taste her, then arched her back for more and brought her pussy closer and closer to Mia's mouth with every hit.

It lasted for 15 minutes until Luke called 'Time Out', and they all repaired to the balcony for more food, drink, a well-deserved rest and a light-hearted conversation, which got Mia's brain in a higher state of bewilderment.

Mia's sexual arousal and curiosity for the forbidden seemed to have overridden any feeling of disgust or unacceptable behaviour and allow her to engage in this sexual activity despite it all willingly.

Three more play sessions, with Luke making passionate love to Sophie, and then he called it a night. No, he hadn't had sex with Mia, but she had enjoyed the experience enormously, but the extraordinary thing was that every time they went out onto the balcony for a break from the sex sessions, they'd talk about politics or business or the environment. Nothing to do with sex and satisfaction. As if it had never taken place.

At the end of the evening, Sophie and Mia kissed Luke good night and went downstairs to dress and leave. Mia was in a state of ecstasy, and her mind was reeling. She'd had some strong orgasms with her interaction with Sophie. She dressed in her street clothes and found her bag by the door.

As she left and walked to her car, she saw that there was a brown envelope in her bag. Sitting in the car, she tore open the envelope, her mind in a whirl, trying to make sense of what had just happened. In the envelope were 15 x $100 notes. $1500! She had just been paid for prostituting herself.

Sitting in the car, parked in a dark laneway, Mia felt wet between her legs and realised that she'd just had a tiny orgasm … alone … thinking about the payment and transaction. She whispered to herself, "What the f**k just happened?"

The essence of Mia's story is transparency and communication between man and woman, or man and man, or woman and woman. Break down the barriers, trust in your partner provided you are in a secure and strong relationship, be open and translucent … and especially don't lie … life would be simpler, more fulfilling, easier and better for us all.

Do people cheat on each other because they have no choice by not having the confidence to speak their mind? Do people divorce because they have no choice? What if we are hurt, because we're not able to communicate each other's hopes and desires rather than by the act of cheating itself? What if we're hurt, not because we've done something wrong, but because we lie about what we did? And all this due to the little fear of been judged by our loved one. Like Mia, her husband's love for her was obviously unconditional, and so he embraced her needs, fantasies and desires.

By changing our perception of 'cheating' as being one big sin and bringing awareness to the core reasons we humans do this. Delving into the taboos of fantasies perhaps is the key to solving what seems to be a huge problem in our society today.

Mia is one of a kind and perhaps she was lucky enough not to have passed the point of no return with her healthy relationship with Rick. I would like to believe that there are a lot of strong, intelligent and secure people out there who can confide in their husbands, wives and partners.

So here's something to think about after such a tale. Do you know who some of the most influential pornographers were in history?

Are you familiar with the names Raphael, Rubens, Michelangelo and Titian? Yes, you guessed it. Some of the greatest painters of the Renaissance and the later periods of art painted nudes on the commission to titillate the taste buds of their patrons.

Throughout the whole of human history, even when we were living in caves, men and women have used sexual objects, toys, idols, pictures, videos and a plethora of other devices, to enhance their sexual responses.

When humans were living in caves, they made sexualised figurines of women, and some of the rock art you see on ancient walls is extremely graphic.

And when the Italian city of Pompeii was excavated in the 1860s, the erotic murals they uncovered shocked such a modest and tight-lipped community. For thousands of years, the Greeks and the Romans were supposed to have been intellectual and sophisticated; but when their art was examined, they saw huge penises and women being penetrated in all sorts of places – I will let you imagine what I mean by that.

So shocked were the Italian authorities that they even banned the public from seeing some of these murals and mosaics, and the 'moveable' objects they found were locked away in a museum in Naples. Of course, nowadays anybody can go to Pompeii and see these wonders of ancient art, but at the time, they gave the Victorians a shock.

Now let's not forget the Hindus of course, with their *Kama Sutra* and all it's erotic drawings. The Ancient Chinese, Thai and Japanese art is also very erotic.

But ever since mankind has been playing with himself … sorry … itself with nudes and eroticism, true pornography, began in the age of Queen Victoria. There were laws in place preventing porn from being sold and distributed. However, it wasn't uncommon for the Victorians to have dirty pictures on their desks at home. And did you know that the dildo was originally a medical instrument developed to bring women to orgasm to rid them of 'mental issues' (most likely believed to be caused by their husbands, who had no idea about how to satisfy a woman)?

In 1959, an enterprising doctor, George Beard, diagnosed these 'medical issues' as 'Hysteria' and began treating such illnesses by providing a gratifying, leg shaking, teeth-clenching orgasm, by placing a dildo where it fit and using his 'medical' skills to provide them with a 'massage' thereby curing them of their Hysteria and making a quick little profit for it.

Another perhaps shocking reality for most is that the electric home vibrator was on the market before many other home appliance essentials; nine years before the electric vacuum cleaner and ten years before the electric iron.

Before we get on with the present situation of pornography and put the past behind us, let's return for a moment to England before the Victorians. The excellent book, *Fanny Hill*, written by John Cleland has subtitled *Memoirs of a Woman of Pleasure*. What a wild read it is. Seriously horny, indelicate, honest and forthright. This book is the most prosecuted and banned book in history, its author and publisher was also prosecuted.

Partly due to the publication of *Fanny Hill*, a group of Victorian worthies calling themselves the Society for the Suppression of Vice tried to get the laws changed to stop all these naughty books, pamphlets, pictures and postcards.

The first known porn film was made in France, where else, at the end of the 19th Century? It was a striptease of a woman called Louise Willy. No, you couldn't invent that if you tried.

Since then, porn has become more and more widely available, up until today it accounts for something like a third of all internet downloads, every second of every day. One-third!

Get this, in 2009; a sex researcher attempted to understand the psychological effects of porn on the human brain by undertaking a study of the way in which pornography alters the minds of men and women. He wanted to find 100 people to participate, 50, who have never watched or been exposed to pornographic material, to take part in the control group, and 50 of whom would need to be regular users. The study was soon to be discontinued because after searching and searching he couldn't find anybody, anybody, who had never been exposed to porn. Now surely that says something about the ubiquity of porn in today's society.

Of course, it's thanks to the Victorians that porn has had such a bad wrap and is today considered to be such a distasteful pastime, enjoyed by horny boys and girls in their teens, and men and women during troubled times in their marriage.

But, in the 19th Century, women who were suffering from continual hysteria went to their doctors, who used dildos on them until they reached orgasm to rid themselves of the 'vapours'. Even today, it's a fact that 75% of women either have never had or rarely have an orgasm. So bring on the dildos.

We began this chapter by calling it 'The Good, the Bad, and the Ugly'.

So what precisely is 'good' about porn?

Well, listening to our mothers and fathers, our teachers and our religious leaders, we'll find that porn is universally wrong. It leads us to bad thoughts and bad ideas, which will lead to sin and destruction (the keyword is a sin). In the old days, we were even told that masturbation led to blindness (of course, if that were true, there wouldn't be too many members of society who have their sight remaining).

We were even taught by our parents that nudity was bad; we were told to put on clothes, and in the age of the Victorians, even little boys and girls weren't allowed to be dressed in comfortable baggy clothes but had to be swaddled in neck to toe outfits that made them look like little men and women. We were told to cover ourselves, and if accidentally, girls showed too much leg or breast in their dresses, they were considered cheap, loose, nasty and whore-ish!

Today, of course, society is much more liberal. Despite some church groups who still make us feel guilty for experiencing pleasure. And in our liberality, especially with the spread of porn on the Internet, an entire industry has grown exponentially, with currently nearly $100 billion (with $12 billion in the United States alone) being spent on it's growth. And no, this is not to say that 'good' business makes 'right' business. Just take a look at the pharmaceutical companies consistently profiting from us.

So the question remains. Is porn good, bad or ugly?

Again, there's not one simple answer, but if you were to consider porn like you do food. It would be easy to see that there is good porn, bad porn, and porn which is not made for consumption.

Good porn is the sort of thing, which individuals, couples or groups can consume on a weekly or less frequent basis (Perhaps something along the lines of Mia and Rick's fantasy). Soft porn can be healthy, sexy, erotic and educational. It can be between men and men, women and women, and men and women, alone or in groups. It can be clothed, naked or in between. It can be spoken or just visual. It is often used to enhance a relationship and explore a little deeper into a partner's desires and fantasies.

So it's not porn per sé which is important, nor the amount, it is rather the type that you chose to watch, and what you're doing while you watch it. If you use porn alone, then a weekly (or perhaps more/less frequent) viewing, leading to an orgasm can relieve stress, tension, and pressure. This way you can focus more without been on edge. Sometimes the pressure is built up in our bodies, and a quickie can be just the right answer. But this needs to be done in private with the right person or hand.

But most importantly, it should not be emotional hidden, covert or under-the-table. If you have a partner and you want to watch porn alone, then share with your partner what you're going to do, or share the experience with them. That alone will relieve the guilt that most people seem to feel when they sneak off and watch porn alone. It all comes from the time when we were children, and our parents told us that sex was a guilty pleasure.

Ok, I understand that it is not easy to tell our partners for the first time we feel the desire to go and watch porn. It will be embarrassing. It perhaps may even lead to the inevitable dreaded question, "Why? Why are you going to do that?"

Be open, honest, and direct. Say, "I want an orgasm, and it's not convenient for you and me to be together right now".

No, it isn't easy, but if you're open, transparent and honest with your partner, then it'll truly make the experience of watching porn far more pleasurable and guilt-free.

What to watch? Well, that's up to you and your personal tastes. But remember that if you watch porn alone and feelings of guilt surround you, the need for more and more porn will always be there. And if there are feelings of guilt attached to watching porn, then it is possible that you will go from an erotic and fun porn experience to a nasty, damagingly fetishistic and harmful experience ... but that's something we'll come to later.

So long, as watching porn is in the balance, in private and you don't hurt anyone or offend anyone, then porn is a terrific sex aid and can lead to a deeper, happier and more understanding relationship with yourself, or with your partner. It can provide an element of novelty into any healthy relationship. Once we make peace with our physiological needs to achieve a happy ending, meaning a good, strong and satisfying orgasm, then porn, used properly, openly and transparently can enhance our sexual desires with our partners and with ourselves. But the operative word is 'transparent'. If porn is hidden, covert and thought of as 'shameful', then it leads to feelings of guilt, which is a sex-killer. I strongly suggest that you discuss your use and desire for porn with your partner. If you don't have a partner, then limit your use of porn to once every now and again maybe once a week, and it'll be all the more satisfying for you.

If you enjoy a variety of what society labels as 'fetishes', such as wearing nylons, pantyhose, older men or women, discipline, high heels, hair, spanking, enemas or the thousand and one other things which turn people on (or off), then there is some great porn on the market, especially the internet. Again, the more open you are with your partner, the more you'll enjoy the fetishes, which turn you on. So there isn't anything in the 'normal' way of sexual turn-ons, which isn't catered for by the Internet. Each and every one can enhance the enjoyment, which you might feel, leading you to a satisfying and guilt free orgasm. The one thing to remember is that you are in control, do not let porn control you.

What does all this mean? Well, in a nutshell, by all means use porn. Alone or with a partner. Use it sparingly like you'd treat yourself to a delicious meal out occasionally. As, like eating fast food every meal of every day, it'll soon become emotionally fattening, and you'll begin to feel yucky. In moderation, when you do use it, relish it like a sex toy, something which brings pleasure, happiness, experience, education and delight to your life then share what you learn with your loved one, and they will appreciate you more for that.

Now let's get onto the 'Bad' and the 'Ugly' part of this Chapter.

This side to porn is that which deals with particular types of unnatural, illegal, inhumane and often even dangerous obsessions. As I've said, we all have fetishes. But there are some who seriously harm the people involved, be recorded without consent and which may even harm the viewer.

But there's also something about the 'bad' and the 'ugly', which is more about the viewer, than by what's being viewed. That is porn addiction.

With those people who are addicted to porn, they usually experience a decline in satisfaction and arousal within their partnership. There's an effect called Coolidge Effect, named after Calvin Coolidge, the President of America in the 1930s. One day,

The President and First Lady were visiting an experimental farm. The First Lady noticed that a rooster was having sex over and over again. She asked how many times he had sex and was told many many times. She said, "Tell that to the President". When President Coolidge watched the same rooster having sex, he asked "Is it always with the same hen?" and was told, "No, Mr. President. With many different hens", to which he replied, "Tell that to Mrs. Coolidge".

The reason I share this with you is that the over-use of porn can lead to not just fewer and less satisfying sexual encounters with your partner but also a desire to have many different partners, putting you in a constant search for freshness, newness and difference. This leads to a lack of intimacy, as we know it. One in five people who regularly watch porn admit to feeling controlled by their sexual desires.

There are some facts, which should concern people who are addicted to porn.

Research shows that such addiction can mean that arousal with a partner declines

Researchers have also found that about half of the people who are trying to give up porn have never had sexual intercourse in their lives, so that their only experience of sex in their lives, and the intimacy which they believe they're going through, is based purely on electronic experiences.

Watching porn these days can begin at the early age of 12, and when adults were asked about their porn habits and history, an alarming 65% said that their tastes in porn had become more and more extreme and had degraded over time, as the 'normal' porn no longer brought them to orgasm.

So here's a bit of good news, 60% of men who give up masturbation and pornography because it's become an obsessive part of their lives, actually report that their sexual functions improve and 67% of men also reported an increase of energy levels as well as productivity when their obsessive masturbation and time spent watching porn was slowed down to a more normal rate of just a couple of times a week.

So let me tell you now about a client of mine who came to see me because he couldn't make love to his partner due to his excessive masturbation. Let's call him David and his partner Anne. Notice how I said 'partner' and not a wife? That's because David was married to a lady whose name is Elizabeth, but she won't play much of a part in this story. Yes, David loved her, but the warmth and sexuality within their marriage just weren't there and hadn't been there for quite some time, so he found Anne.

David and his wife Elizabeth hadn't had sex for years and years ... and years. Perhaps this sounds all too familiar right? The physically intimate aspect of their life had evaporated from their marriage after the birth of their children. David was a very busy filmmaker, and his wife Elizabeth was a university lecturer. They led incredibly hectic and fruitful lives, but after their children had been born, their careers became increasingly frantic, and they were travelling more and more, alone he, to Hollywood and on locations and she, to conferences and mentorships.

As their sex lives devolved, and through frustration, David began masturbating to Internet porn until, dissatisfied, he joined a pay-for-sex dating site.

Well, on this dating and paying site, he met Anne. She was a match, and so they arranged to meet for an Italian meal in a restaurant in the south of the city where they lived.

It certainly wasn't love at first sight. Anne was there to enter into a win-win arrangement, and he was there to pay for someone to take his frustration away. As it wasn't a prostitution service, they met as boyfriend and girlfriend. And both, being in their adult years weren't expecting love, just friendship, sex and enjoyment. It was a designer relationship. She adored his intellect and artistic nature; he adored her brains, her humour, her wild-eyed approach to life, and her sexiness ... oh boy, did he enjoy her sexiness ... Ultimately it was love that they found.

Their first lunch took them over three hours; they talked, laughed, and drank. He experienced the warmth of a woman that he hadn't known since the early years of his relationship with Elizabeth.

Both David and Anne enjoyed each other so much that when they left, they walked down to the car park arm in arm, once he was sat in the driver's seat of his car, ready to go Anne didn't say goodbye, she instead walked around the car and hopped into the passenger's seat. Surprised, David looked at her, and without a word, she reached across and started to massage his lap.

He'd never experienced anything like it before, except in the fantasy world of pornography where such things happened all the time.

Was Anne a porn star? No, she was an entirely open, sexual, transparently attractive and gorgeous woman who was at peace with her body and her mind. She was attracted to David's brains and body and wanted him to take away the same joyous memories that she was going to take away from their first meeting.

So just like that in the car park, in public, and for David's first ever experience, she reached over and kissed him. She pulled down the zipper of his pants and kissed him in a place where his wife Elizabeth hadn't visited in years.

He couldn't put Anne out of his mind from that moment onwards. She was his every waking thought, and she dominated his life. Sure, he continued to work, and his relationship with his wife Elizabeth was just as it had been. He went to bed thinking about Anne. Woke thinking about her, and was thinking about her when he made his wife a cup of peppermint tea, as he did every night.

They met again and again, and it wasn't long before he was in her bed. His performance was woeful because of the anxiety he felt after all those years of not making love to a woman, and only masturbating to porn on the Internet. So he wasn't able to function, and Anne became frustrated because he couldn't get it sufficiently rigid to enter her. But with his mouth and fingers, he satisfied her. And he was able to orgasm well enough.

Later that day, he returned home, and went onto the Internet to watch porn, and came strongly, closing his eyes instead of watching the actors and actresses making love. With his eyes shut, he thought of Anne and her body, her beautiful black hair, her glorious blue eyes and her incredible white skin. He came so vigorously and loudly that Elizabeth, in another part of his house, shouted out and asked him if he was alright.

He and Anne met many times subsequently, but he was still unable to function sexually. So he came clean with Anne and admitted to watching porn, telling her that he couldn't stop. At first, she was insulted, wanting to know why he couldn't get sufficiently rigid to enter her body, yet was very stiff when watching some 'Hollywood Bimbo' pretending to enjoy sex.

So on her advice, he sought help ... my help.

I advised him of the joys and wonders of occasional masturbation, especially with a partner; but I also warned him of the very real dangers of covert and excessive masturbation and addiction to pornography.

He took my advice. He told Anne, and together they began to watch and enjoy porn, but not excessively; only on occasions. Afterwards or sometimes even during their porn watching, they would spend time caressing each other, playing and massaging one another sensually. It took David six months to get back close to physically responding to Anne's body again and only then he started enjoying the benefits of a more happy relationship with his lover in an environment where his exposure to porn was more controlled and less controlling.

As they watched, she performed for him what the actresses were doing to their male counterparts; this was something which his wife Elizabeth would never have considered doing. As for his part, he returned the favour and performed on Anne like a Hollywood porn star.

Now he and Anne are both happy, and so is Elizabeth. Why? Well, due to David stopping his addiction to porn, he and Elizabeth have been able to reconnect with each other on a physical level, and they have never been happier.

Fidelity, or rather, infidelity, is not something of importance to either of them, but a more fulfilled sexual life is. And with this new regimen, David is a lot more content within himself, his relationships and his sexuality; and Elizabeth is content with the occasional cuddle, with a cold 'good night kiss' and that is as far as they will get physically with to each other.

As a practitioner and after seeing these issues time and time again and understanding the stress that such experiences impose not only on David's emotional, his physical and mental bodies but also on their relationship. It makes me wonder whether monogamy is a normal and realistic expectation for some of us?

Did watching porn harm his marriage? No, he still has a riotous sex life with Anne, what porn has done in David's marriage is enhance his love and friendship with his wife, Elizabeth. I told him to carefully consider the need and the potential consequences of telling Elizabeth what he'd been up to with Anne. Wives will appreciate transparency, but it will take someone incredibly balanced and secure within their relationship to accept infidelity, in my view what the appropriate thing to do is entirely up to the individual. The way in which our society has conditioned us to accept the truth of religion and an imposed set of moral principles allows marriages to go on (perhaps turning a blind eye) even when the suspicion of infidelity is there between us, causing an unspoken tension and strife in our marriage. A lot of us put up with it, knowing entirely well that we may not bring enough to fulfil our partner in all the ways they need to be fulfilled.

So the question which has to be asked, and which will shock many readers is simply this … why should a man or woman suffer because the other partner withdraws from an active sex life? A temporary withdrawal is one thing, but a permanent withdrawal, which is far more widespread than most people think, is unjust, unfair, and damaging. Many older couples have sex once a month, sometimes once every six months. And many don't have sex any longer, citing impotence, disinterest, exhaustion or illness.

But is it fair to the other partner? And how long should a partner be expected to be in a state of frustration without resorting to masturbating with pornography, or visiting a prostitute, or having a paramour?

Those are questions which only the individuals can answer, but one day, the churches will accept that their millennia-old prohibition of any form of relationship other than monogamy (and no sex before marriage) is outmoded, arbitrary, wrong and damaging.

CHAPTER SIX

The Joys and Oys, of being single

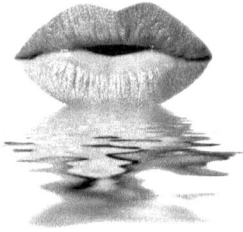

Being single doesn't mean you're weak. It means you're strong enough to wait for what YOU deserve.

Most of us live our lives in a community. It could be a community of two, four, or more; it could be a community in our homes where your partner and your children are there to support and be a part of your life. Some of us have a much wider community, such as in our professional lives, or we're members of a club or association.

Whatever community we're part of, we often rely heavily on family and friends to extend us beyond ourselves. We are in part, a reflection of those who know and love us.

But some people, through their volition or circumstance, don't have a broad community. Some live alone through not finding a life-partner, or through divorce or death; some people, especially older ones, live in their home and rarely step out onto the pavement to join the rivers of people going backwards and forwards in their lives.

Social isolation has an enormous impact in our community and amongst those who suffer from it are people who have travelled far and settled from another country. Refugees, asylum seekers, are often bereft of companionship, and seek solace in those upon whom they know from their communities.

But it doesn't end there; we also have hundreds of other little things that contribute to our isolation, the endless hours we are spending sitting in traffic these days, the extended hours we are working, not to mention some hours we devote to the Internet. We seem to have a long list of justifications not to connect with other people physically, and this is turning us into a sick society unlike any which has ever previously existed. It's making us ill, and the isolation is causing an epidemic of mental and physical illnesses. And this is being called an epidemic? Yes, social isolation is a growing menace as we live our lives in separation from others, separated by machines, with a lack of human contact, the destruction of old neighbourhoods, and the increasing population working from their homes.

There was a time where we humans lived together in tribes, clans, and neighbourhoods. The foundation unit was the family. Today, this complex society of networks is breaking down, and so are we.

We humans are just not designed to live like this. It is not in our DNA. We originated as hunter-gatherer communities that spent most of the time in groups with families and loved ones. The men went out hunting, while those left behind gathered, and prepared jointly, the things, which were needed for survival. It was an all day, every day relationship.

Is it possible that without even realising it we are choosing to replace deep friendships with screens, gadgets and endless hours binging Netflix shows? Do we fully comprehend the harm we are inflicting upon ourselves?

It's these people who are the subject of this chapter in my book. Because there are unique issues to consider about living a life alone.

On the one hand, there are very real benefits – though they might not seem apparent immediately, especially in the early stages of being alone.

These could involve total independence (particularly after a lifetime of being dependent on another person), nearly 44% of people over 65 live alone and of this group 69% are women, as statistically speaking women tend to outlive their male counterparts. Your personal space has suddenly increased whether or not you like it, and you are free to do as you please, be organised or not, get out of bed when you want, or stay there under the blankets. You can choose your décor for your entire place, you can finally enjoy some peace and quiet, you can cook whatever you feel like and your food can be as aromatic and spicy as you like it, and when the spicy food aggressively leaves your body ... well, there is no one there to make a sarcastic comment about the smell.

But on the other hand, there is a popular saying that man is a social animal and this by far is the significant disadvantage of living alone, which might not seem immediately apparent, but which could involve illness, disease, mental problems and failure to connect at a deep level.

Loneliness is one of the principal causes of suicide and is increasingly being recognised as a cause of devastating complaints that range from such issues as anxiety, high blood pressure, and depression. And of course there are exceptions to these rules, but we are not going to measure the rules by the minority of people that wouldn't think twice about living their lives all on their own and be euphoric and healthy with it.

There is also a very real causal link between a person's relationship status and their wellbeing. The divorce rate according to some researchers is in the vicinity of 50%. Although there is a minority of this group of divorcees who move quite rapidly onto the next relationship, for the majority of people the phase after divorce means time out and sometimes people never remarry or form a steady relationship.

Some of us, by no deliberation, tend to sabotage any possibility of a new relationship with isolation, in order to recover from a wounded soul or even draw in the pain or sorrow of a previous relationship. These individuals often do absolutely nothing to let go of the pain and improve their state of being. We can also choose to use this time to get to know exactly what it is we want in life; the likes and dislikes and to deeply get to know ourselves and find our roots again.

In any case, one thing rings true If you're in your early 40s or 50s, then your health will improve by your being more active. This isn't always the case, of course, but look at the reality. If you're in your 40s and like 50% of the population, you go through a divorce or separation you are still young enough to want to find another partner (hopefully this next one is better than the previous). So you go jogging, or to the gym, or lift weights or go on a diet to revive the body you had when you were 25.

So being suddenly single in your 40s or 50s could be emancipation (after the devastation), and life could very well take on a whole new meaning.

But if you're older, say in your 60s, 70s or 80s, then the chances of finding another life partner are considerably slimmer.

We've all seen films from America about cruise boats floating around the Caribbean in which old matrons were weighing upwards of 90 kilos go to the gym of the ship and proceed to make flirting noises at every man who passes.

Well, that's Hollywood. In real life, if you've passed the age of

70, the chances of finding a second life with somebody is marginal at best.

Which means that at these ages, we have to concern ourselves with health and wellbeing on the assumption that you won't have somebody with you into the future.

LONELINESS, WELLBEING and THE Third Age

The ageing population is expected to increase over the coming years. It is also expected that the number of people over 80 is going to double by 2037 and loneliness is going to be a major concern for older people. I will refer to this as our Fourth Age, *Looking into the Fourth Age* is another one of my books. Let's just say this is a very sensitive subject, that people who reach this age often suffer from the lack of desire and affection, that there is not enough closeness and or social interaction and some of this will bring with it a desire to end some people's life on earth in some cases. As a baby boomer, we owe it to ourselves and the future generations to do something about this and raise awareness, and we will.

Yes, there are some personal and even social benefits to living alone, especially after living in a claustrophobic relationship, which was destructive and damaging to you and your partner.

You can walk around the house without any clothes on. You can reheat food, and even have a multiplicity of lovers if that is what you wish. You can cook the meals that you want to eat. You can flick the channel as many times as you want to and even watch movies, which your ex wouldn't allow you to watch. These are the good things. But we have to look at the bad things as well.

What are the disadvantages of being alone, especially regarding wellness?

The most obvious is loneliness. And loneliness isn't just being alone, not having somebody to talk to, going to bed and waking up in the morning, and finding the lounge room and kitchen in the same state as you left it, having nobody to take care of you, bringing you a cup of coffee in the morning. But loneliness goes much deeper than the surface meaning of not having somebody for cuddles in bed.

Loneliness is when you feel emotionally and socially disconnected. It doesn't matter how many friends or relatives who live close by. Loneliness suppresses the functioning of your immune system.

Loneliness, according to medical science, is as damaging to one's health as smoking 15 cigarettes a day, with older generations in as much danger of ill health as younger migrants being forced to move overseas. Social isolation among older people, 65 and over, puts ageing populations at a higher risk of dementia, cardiovascular disease, and decreased immune system responses.

Loneliness is also an aspect of our self-esteem. When you're alone, you miss knowing that you're loved. Not just having nobody to share thoughts and feelings with, but knowing every day that your hopes and aspirations, doubts and fears, frustrations and desires will always be locked inside of you.

It can lead to feeling secluded from society as if you're adrift on a pedestrian island in the middle of the street, watching crowds of people on the pavements walking, talking and laughing. You just want to scream out 'Hey! Look at me! I'm a good person ... come over here and talk to me'.

And unfortunately, because partnerships and couples dominate so much of Western society, marriages and relationships, a person who lives life alone, is often looked down upon, by friends and colleagues. Some will show concern and yet won't include you in anything they organise, or perhaps continually try to set you up with 'a great guy', just because you are on your own.

If you work all day in an office or a shop, and when your friends and colleagues tell you what they and their families are having for dinner that night, you'll catch them looking at you in compassion. And often, you'll take that look as 'pity', and you'll be offended.

One of the problems, which an older person experiences when alone, is a decline in physical activity it seems that the lonely and single version of ourselves is not worth the effort and so we neglect our bodies, the basis of existence. Moving is one of the most important parts of keeping our bodies in the balance, with a partner, you're more inclined to do things, go out for walks, go to places together, experience the new scenery, maybe go to a sports ground and do gentle exercises. But when you're suddenly alone – by way of divorce or death – it's just so easy to stay at home, cook yourself a meal, watch TV, go to bed and think about your condition of loneliness. But there is a way to alleviate the difficulties of isolation, at least on a physical level, and it'll do more than just that, it'll give you more confidence, and probably introduce you to a range of new people who'll share your interests,

How?

By increasing your physical activity when you've just been left alone (death or divorce?), the last thing you want to do is to pound the pavement and work up a sweat. But when you've been alone for a while – it's entirely up to you to determine when you should do it – there will come a time when you'll want to get out of the house and back into society.

One way of breaking down the wall, which is preventing you from making that first step, is to go out and walk for fifteen minutes or a half an hour. Go to the shops, go to the park, go along the main road or a side street ... but just go.

You'll find that your pulse rate will increase, you'll flush and feel sweaty, and when you've returned home and drunk that mandatory glass of water, you'll feel so much better.

But here's the important thing.

Tomorrow, at about the same time, do the same thing again but chose a different route. Persistence will help to break up the routine, and you'll want to go out on subsequent days and find new ways and paths on which to walk.

Do this regularly, every day if possible, and in a week when it's becoming a habit treat yourself to a pair of runners, or some new walking clothes. This way you will keep motivated to continue creating this habit of yours, and you'll continue integrating it into your life.

So what are the advantages of doing this? Well, the main benefit is that its gentle exercise, which will benefit your cardiovascular health. It's good for your weight, your chest, and your morale.

It'll help you lose weight, keep you fit and make you feel much better within yourself.

But there's another massive advantage that will happen.

As you exercise on a regular basis, you'll become a part of a different society from the one in which you traditionally live. When we're recently alone, we tend to come to rely on family, sons and daughters, sisters, uncles and aunts and good friends.

But as the months and years wear on, we tend to restrict our circle of friends, until we realise that there are only a few who are close to us. So we need to get out into a new circle of people to revitalise our place in society. We delay this and put it off for fear of uncertainty and insecurity.

The problem with being alone, though, is that most of us become introvert and unwilling to take the (self-perceived and probably fictional) risk of opening ourselves up to new people. And that fear of belonging, which we all feel at some point in life, is ignited, again and again, so we don't accept our differences, but part of us just wants to fit in and belong to a group, to society, to people, instinctively thinking that that will make us happy. We spend years upon years trying to figure out a way to be part of, without realising that the multitude shares those exact feelings, that we are not alone that there are other lonely people out there. Even as adults we tend to gravitate towards people we think we fit in with and sometimes instead of hanging in there and pushing past the discomfort of not fitting in we just flee the scene and head back to our forte, the safety and comfort of our home.

But, and this is a fabulous but, when we branch out on our own into a society of other people who are doing things alone; like walking, jogging or working out in the gym. We see them pushing through the fear of not belonging and only then within a few days of regular visits or seeing the same people, we make eye contact, smile, nod and say 'How are you?'. From then on, it evolves and gradually develops into a friendship, simply because you made the decision to get out of the house.

That is one major way of overcoming loneliness and immersing yourself into a new society. It takes all of us to make a community, and you are a paramount part of it because you count!

LONELINESS WITHIN A PARTNERSHIP

But it's not only people who are not in a relationship, marriage or partnership that can be lonely. It's a statistical fact that 60% of lonely people are married.

Let me say that again, nearly two-thirds of all married men and women are lonely. Alone. Without intimacy and often feeling insecure. Unsure of themselves and their position within the relationship with a sense of disassociation from their partners.

Just because a couple is in a relationship, it doesn't for one moment mean that they're not lonely. Loneliness, in this case, isn't companionship. It isn't referring to when one partner is off fishing for the day, while the other stays at home cooking and tending to the children.

It doesn't mean that one is off with another person, while the other is sitting at home with a box of Kleenex and a carton of ice cream.

Loving partners, good friends, those who spend most evenings and mornings together, can be intensely lonely within their relationship.

What's missing, and what causes the intense frustrations of loneliness, is the bond of intimacy. Through the years we seem to take each other for granted, I heard a friend of mine saying to me the other day "I was in my late forties, three kids, a lovely house, two cars, a great job, but no sex. I wasn't going anywhere, of course; we had a sexless matrimony but who cares ..."

So again, what is intimacy? And why is it missing, and absent, from nearly two-thirds of all relationships?

Intimacy is the glue, which keeps a relationship fresh, alive, close and together, intimacy is not only physical, it's emotional, social, mental, and when you have it in any relationship it is so rewarding. So how do we achieve intimacy? Through transparent communication; with the extraordinary ability to communicate our thoughts and feelings to another person, without the fear of being judged. Unfortunately, in this society, this is something, which seldom exists.

So is communication the be all and end all? Is communication the key to an intimate and loving relationship? Absolutely.

Not just communicating "What's on TV tonight"?' or "A letter arrived for you".

But communicating with intimacy our hopes, desires, concerns, frustrations and fears.

If a partner likes to be touched, to be spoken to in a certain way, then communication is the way to making it happen. If not, then a lack of empathy and understanding of the other's needs, will lead to frustration, alienation and the worst of all these emotions, resentment.

One of my clients had a strong desire to make love to his wife while she was wearing sheer black stockings. But he was too shy to ask her, fearing her ridicule and rejection, and so he said nothing, this led to a build up in his frustration, which turned to resentment towards her and their relationship. Until one day, he was with a co-worker, who loved wearing black stockings, he took this opportunity and made a sexual advance towards her and they began an affair, which led to the breakup of his marriage. Was his divorce preventable? Maybe.

FOMO – FEAR OF MISSING OUT

Fear of missing out is one of the reasons for loneliness. Sometimes, we sabotage our relationships because of FOMO; fear of missing out on what could be a relationship because of our concerns that there could be an even better, sexier, more intimate relationship around the corner.

Take this client of mine who tracked down and reconnected with his first love on Facebook. She was happily married to her current husband. Yet, those Facebook adventures lead her to have an affair with her 'young love' because she thought they belonged together. She forgot why they broke up in the first place, and wanted to feel what it was like to be that young girl and boy once more.

Her husband could not forgive her and thereby requested a divorce. Certainly, there is more to this ending than just the affair, but there weren't any lines open for communication, she used this as her way out, from what they had seemed to have settled with a happy but mediocre, non-exciting life of togetherness.

When we're in a state of a non-relationship, when we're alone and, like Keat's knight in *La Belle Dame Sans Merci*, 'We're on our own and palely loitering', we look forward to meeting somebody who will promise to fill in the gaps we have created in our lives.

If fortune smiles on us and we meet somebody or simply reconnect with someone from the past, knowing that there was a reason for the separation in the first instance, there are many people who will not allow the relationship to develop. Most of us will understand that this relationship no longer ticks all the boxes, which it once did in our youth and we will feel that there is another person, yet 'to cross our path, who is more 'right' for us.

In life today, we're exposed to so many different people, especially through the Internet. It has become so easy to meet people via electronic and social media, and this has made us uncertain of settling for just one because our landscapes are incredibly full of people who could make all the difference to our lives.

In a recent survey, it was found that adults spent 2.1 hours a day on social media platforms; but in comparison, teenagers were spending 2.7 hours a day. So the differences between what time adults spend and kids spend talking to people in the hope of furthering a relationship, is minimal.

Looking at the adult population, almost one person in four reported being heavy social media users, and 6% of those admitting to being continuously connected. So social media is both a cause and a means of managing, stress. Both adults and teens experience this new found, 'Fear Of Missing Out'.

The relationship between excessive social media use and FOMO, we found, is that teens are more likely to experience more aspects of fear of missing out, than are adults. What this indicates is that social media has a greater impact on teens, and therefore is more aligned to their identity and their search for a sense of self.

So are we better to be in a marriage, partnership or relationship, which is unhappy, with the hope of it potentially, getting better, or are we better off separating? And if we do stay in the relationship, we have to ask ourselves, why? Why do we put up with the trauma, the continual unhappiness, tension, frustration and heartache, when it's so simple these days to separate?

There's no right or wrong answer. Each person has his or her reasons for staying in a relationship, or for leaving.

Perhaps the best way to define an answer is to talk about one of my clients, and his relationship, and the reason that, after 39 years of marriage, some of it happy, most of it sad – frustrating and sad – he decided after consultations with me, to remain.

Let's call him Tom. He met and married Clair when he was working as a musician in New York, and she was visiting on holiday. They met in a bar, started to chat, and within two days, she'd moved out of her hotel, and into his apartment. Within a week of hothouse living, loving and being entertained by the enormity of the city and what it could provide, they'd decided to marry, and arranged a trip back to their homes. Fortunately, they came from the same town, so it was all very convenient.

Within a year, they were married, and living blissfully at home. Tom was very successful as a musician, and Clair was a university lecturer in botany and was studying for her doctorate.

The marriage quickly produced two glorious children. It really couldn't have been a happier marriage. They had beautiful professional lives, a gorgeous family, lots of friends, and were already being noted in the media. No, nothing went wrong. But because of their love for each other, their relationship changed, slowly and subtly, but inexorably. They were no longer independent people, no longer individuals, but became co-dependent. Tom depended on Clair for advice, assistance, understanding, warmth and love; Clair depended on Tom to support her in the house when she was giving an evening lecture, to help with the kids.

Soon, they were no longer husband and wife, but each other's carers. And this didn't mean that love disappeared from the marriage, but that the love transmuted into a different form. It was more of a parental love than matrimonial. Although we are all multi-dimensional beings in relationships, and that all relationships should be established from the balance of the multidimensional being we are.

What tends to happen in most marriages is that we find comfort within a couple of those multifaceted acts and so some become purely sexual, and there's no other type of intimacy, and for others, it's only friendship, and they concentrate on these strengths. For some, it's just parental.

Fine tuning the will is hard to do unless you're a whole balanced being. But when you lose yourself in a 'one plus one equals two' relationship, as opposed to 'three', then it becomes a co-dependent relationship. And this is precisely what had happened to Tom and Clair. The longer they left it, the harder it was for either of them to establish 'wholeness' within themselves.

Neither Tom nor Clair recognised it, of course, each, thinking that they were still an ideal husband and wife in a perfect marriage. But the reality was that, as she looked on him as her back up, her best friend, and he looked upon her as the same, the sexual side of their marriage became less intimate and slowly dissipated.

In this new role as co-dependents, they continued to make love, but it was more by way of physical release than the deep intimacy they'd once felt. And after many more years, the lovemaking dropped from twice a week, to twice a month, to almost never.

He would be in his office, writing musical compositions, and when he was exhausted, go to bed when she was almost asleep. He'd undress quietly, and crawl into bed beside her. Then she'd wake, turn and kiss him goodnight. Then turn around and go back to sleep. He would remain awake for some time, wondering why life was passing him by.

This situation lasted for another twelve years. There was no unhappiness in the marriage, no anger, no shouting. However, by a similar token, there was no romance, no intimacy, and certainly no closeness, which wasn't akin to friendship.

If they made love, it was because Tom begged Clair. And when they did, he could sense that she was just waiting for it to be over so that she could return to researching her plants.

Which was when Tom came to see me. He told me that he was thinking of leaving Clair. The kids were now old enough to move out of home into their apartments, and he was in his late 50s and still young enough to find another wife.

But his problem was that he was feeling intensely guilty because he knew that it would destroy Clair; that it would be so unexpected, and so antipathetic to their friendship, that she'd think he'd had a brain seisure.

He asked me what he should do? Should he leave an unhappy marriage, and strive to find happiness, or should he stay married, and find a mistress, he felt stuck on what was the right thing to do.

But no matter how desperate he was for advice, I refused to give it. I wasn't going to tell him what he should do. This was an answer which would have to come from him, his conscience, his heart, and his understanding of his situation that he found himself in.

So we sat for a long, long time and talked about how his once loving marriage had devolved into a one plus one equals two co-dependency when it had started off as a one plus one equals three synergies. So I drew up a list for Tom, and we spent a couple of hours working it through. It's a list I often use with clients who think that everything is perfect and can't see the reality of the relationship. This will unveil where his actual relationship status was with Clair.

I showed him the list, and so he filled in the blanks, and this is something, which anybody could do. It is a total eye-opener.

WHEN I FEEL RESPONSIBLE IN A RELATIONSHIP …

For Others

- [ ] I fix
- [ ] I protect
- [ ] I rescue
- [ ] I control
- [ ] I carry their feelings
- [ ] I don't listen
- [ ] I feel tired
- [ ] I feel anxious
- [ ] I feel fearful
- [ ] I feel liable
- [ ] I am concerned with solutions
- [ ] I am concerned with answers
- [ ] I am concerned with circumstances
- [ ] I am concerned with being right
- [ ] I am concerned with details
- [ ] I am concerned with being performance

To Others

- [ ] I show understanding and compassion
- [ ] I share
- [ ] I challenge
- [ ] I level
- [ ] I am sensitive
- [ ] I attentive
- [ ] I feel relaxed
- [ ] I feel free
- [ ] I feel aware
- [ ] I feel good about myself
- [ ] I am concerned with relating one to one
- [ ] I am concerned with feelings
- [ ] I am concerned with the person

It took Tom some time to tick off the list. At first, he found it confronting and challenging because even though it looks deceptively simple, it's something which gets to the very heart of our personalities.

This is a great thing for you, or anybody to do, especially if you're in a relationship that seems to be stable, but still hanging by a thread.

Look at the list, and tick those boxes which you consider apply to you. Ask your partner to do the same.

And then, sit down and discuss it. On the following, you'll find the answer to where you are as an individual, and as part of the relationship, This is the very core of the relationship and your place within it.

If you've ticked more of the left column than the right, then read the comments on the left-hand side of the columns below.

If you ticked more of the right-hand column, then refer to the comments on the right-hand side of the comments below.

The ideal way to improve where you're tendencies are, is to work towards the right-hand side of the comments.

I am a manipulator	I believe if I just share myself, the other person has enough to make it
I am an egoist	I like a win-win situation
I expect the person to live up to my expectations	I am a helper and guide
I'm only happy when I'm in control. 'm unhappy when somebody else takes the decisions	I expect the person to be responsible to him/herself and his actions
I want to know what my partner is doing	I can trust and let go
I prefer to keep myself to myself	I can be honest and transparent

So when Tom ticked far more of the left-hand side of the columns than the right-hand side, and I showed him the comments which showed him the second list which outlines his personality characteristics, he was stunned.

But once I'd talked it through with him, it soon became apparent that his marriage, far from being irreparable, was fixable. What he had to do was to allow Clair to be herself, not to protect her, not to attempt to live her life for her, and to be more of a husband than a father figure. He recognised that he had to bring more of the multidimensional aspects of his personality to the marriage to achieve balance into their relationship. But it wasn't that simple because he had to get Clair to read the list, and recognise that she was as much part of the solution, as she was part of the problem. It was important that they both shared credit as they changed and did not blame or avoided to claim responsibility.

People do need people no matter what, no matter where we need to accept that we are not created equal and must respect other's feelings and respect each other enough to listen is the key to a successful relationship.

Whether you decide to be on your own or with someone else you must understand and use the necessary tools you have on hand. You owe it to yourself to find 'wholeness' and a sense of 'responsibility' within everything you do. Be clear in what you want, take full responsibility for your actions and ask when in doubt. Find new strategies to shift the paradigms that are not allowing you to regularly achieve growth in your health and wellness. Don't give up on yourself get out there and leave an imprint.

Do something different every day, learn a new word, take yourself to the movies yes on your own if you have to, it's quite an empowering feeling.

Find a group of people that have similar ideas of what fun is. Sydney meetups is a great way to meet other mind-liked people.

Humans have the tendency to repeat behaviours and thoughts every day; this is a habitual and unconscious action.

So challenge yourself and for the next 30 days try doing something new, here is a list for you to add on, to suit your likes:

1. Walk to the shops through a different route.
2. Brush your teeth with the opposite hand for on every second day.
3. Sing yourself a lullaby before you go to bed.
4. Go to bed earlier than normal.
5. Sleep on the other side of the bed.
6. Write a blog, an article.
7. Take a class to learn painting, creative writing or another language.
8. Join a gym.
9. Join a yoga class.
10. Don't complain for a day.
11. Say "Hi" to a complete stranger.
12. Pay a coffee forward.
13.
14.
15.
16.
17.
18.
19.
20.
21.
22.
23.
24.
25.
26.
27.
28.
29.
30.

When filling these in think of all the simple things that will connect you to at least one other person and encourage human interaction. You will meet new people and discover great things about yourself that maybe you have never known before or perhaps deep down you knew but you were just afraid to tap into.

CHAPTER SEVEN

Are men in this alone?

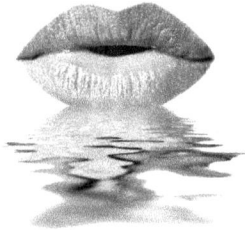

Challenge your limiting beliefs about masculinity such as 'Men are always in control' or 'Boys don't cry'.

Here's a serious question. And it's addressed to every man reading this. No, not my women readers. This chapter is for men only!

So gentlemen, read on.

Do you remember the last time you had an orgasm? When you made love to a partner and reached that wondrous bodily point where no matter what, you have to keep going and keep going and keep ah. You know what I mean. You had an intense orgasm. Your penis grew that little bit longer, you ran to the top of your physical and emotional cliff, and when you were just at the very summit, it came, and you jumped over the top of the cliff and launched yourself into free, open air, into space, into a landscape of utter joy.

Remember? We've all done it, either alone, with a partner or with many different partners.

Please stay with that thought; I'm ONLY talking to men. So ... now do you remember?

Good!

Then think beyond your reaction, your orgasm. Your moment of sexual climax. Think about what happened just before you rolled off, or from under your lover, and lay on the bed, the couch, the mound of grass or the cliff top, and breathed in deeply and felt your body suffused with the warmth and joy of a post-coital orgasmic release.

Think about that moment, just before your orgasm! Right.

Let's stop here for a moment, before I ask you a very crucial question. Let's see what happens physically to men during sex according to two of my clients.

Tim, mid 40s works in IT said that during sex he gets like in a trance, and although he's physically present, his mind wanders into the horny realms of out of space, he says it's very hard to explain. Once he comes for a second, his entire body is in a state of bliss, and it is as if the colours are brighter and his senses are heightened, he also admits that the intensity of his orgasms varies depending on how long he holds out for.

Robert (52 years old), is an accountant and he challenges himself to hold back on his orgasms for as long as he can to make them more intense, after some practice he has noticed a big difference between "just letting go" and controlling the urge. But after he reaches a point of no return and finally cums he feels hazy and spaced out and quite often he just drift into a sleep.

So I would like to ask you what does your orgasmic experience feel like? I want you to stop reading for a second and try to imagine that moment.

Now think about your partner! Did she have an orgasm? Did you feel her vagina squeeze your penis in a series of contractions? Did you feel her chest suddenly heave? Did you feel the warmth of her wetness? Did she suddenly hug you and hold you close as her body was swamped with her building up to reach climax?

And if you don't remember the answers to any of these questions, tell me, did you ask her if she reached an orgasm before you let go of yours? Did you stare into her eyes, see her lips moist, feel her breath suddenly quicken, her hands suddenly grasp your body?

And if you didn't ask her whether she'd had an orgasm, did you ask yourself whether or not you should or could now do something to bring her to the same state of unutterable peace and satisfaction as you're enjoying?

Sorry if these questions have discombobulated you and thrown you out of balance. If they've made you feel just a tiny bit guilty and selfish.

However, according to Planned Parenthood statistics, as many as 1 in 3 women have trouble reaching orgasm when engaging in intercourse. And as many as 80%, of women, have difficulty with orgasm from vaginal stimulation alone. Clitoral stimulation during intercourse often helps. So guys although it is true that women when they reach orgasm, seem to be experiencing a much more powerful climax than you … please know that it is harder for them to get there and so they need your help.

My suggestions to you are to ensure that she is ready for intercourse/penetration and that means foreplay, 2 minutes is not enough time typically required for women to get to a point where penetration is enjoyable. As a general rule of thumb, I would recommend sticking to no less than 10 to 15 minutes of foreplay. Please do keep in mind that this is a general guidance and that all women are different. So do your due diligence and find out what she prefers or needs before she is ready.

Making love is an art. Sometimes you are inspired, and things flow naturally but other times you have both got to work at it a little more. By learning the tools of intimacy and showing some respect and asking questions, rather than just assuming, your willingness to please your lover will show your tenderness, and they will see how you care about all aspects of what makes her wet. This way when you surface the edge of pleasure, you will have created a great, safe space for the both of you to enjoy it as much as each other.

But that's the problem with so many marriages, especially as men and women reach their middle age. It tends to lead towards a breakdown in communication, long-term frustration for the man's lover, and in many cases, a split in the marriage. Does this only happen in later life? No, it can occur at any stage, to anyone, and indeed all the way through from the honeymoon period of a relationship to having a long history together. However, one thing they all have in common is that it is a cause for intense resentment.

One lady I know, in her middle age, has just met a new boyfriend, and they have great sex together. He reaches climax and has an intense orgasm whenever they are together which she willingly assists him within the many varied ways that he profoundly enjoys to reach his peak. Once he has cum, he rolls over and goes to sleep. She asks him, why he left her half way up the hill and without bringing her to a complete state of satisfaction, and he is surprised. He responds with "I thought you had an orgasm". And she asks him, "Did you ask?, You just assumed, and when you assume, you made an ass of you and me". He was a little shocked.

She adores him. He adores her, but their relationship is on the rocks because he's only looking after his sexual needs. This is a trait that is quite typical of an alpha male.

But where does it all start? Is it a function of middle age, or does it plant it's roots earlier in life? The answer may surprise you.

From the many hundreds of clients I've spoken to about this issue, I've come to the conclusion that it begins in childhood. When the boy is growing up, if his parents have trained him to respect other people, if they have instilled in him the morals to be an empathetic individual when it comes to other people's feelings, like giving and sharing without feeling jealous, and ensuring that his happiness is shared, then this is the sort of upbringing ensures that he grows up making sure that he has a lover who is satisfied, and that is one of the foundations that will hold a relationship together. It's not so much himself that he is concerned about, it is more about the happiness that he feels when giving and sharing and allowing his partner to feel the same sense of satisfaction that he is receiving. It's these little things in a child's upbringing, which can make such a huge difference in a man's later life.

So let's look at the opposite case. A boy who is brought up to acknowledge and adopt all of the traditional machos, masculine things which heroes are suppose to adopt – stoicism, winning at all costs, and coming second has no place in success – he is a kid who'll grow up not to have an appreciation of another person feelings, needs or wants.

When this young boy finally marries, it will be his decisions that count; it will be his wife who will always play the role of the subordinate; and worse, much worse, it will be him who reaches orgasm first, and whether his wife climaxes or not is of less importance to him.

At the beginning of this book, we talked about intimacy. What is intimacy again? Intimacy is the experience of emotional closeness, Oh No! Stop right there! Emotional closeness? It is widely known that this is something, which so many men avoid at all costs.

From childhood, we teach our sons very different morals than those we teach our daughters. We teach girls to share, to be considerate, to please others and to say yes. But what do we teach boys? Well, and this is a generalisation, we tend to teach them from an earlier age not to show emotions, not to cry, to be 'a man', not to show their real feelings and emotions, and worse, much worse, that 'real men' are sexual aggressors, and that to admit fear, discomfort or confusion about sex implies some level of vulnerability. Oh no, there is that word again vulnerable!

There are different aspects of their sexual desires that we teach our sons, and almost all of them have quite a detrimental impact, on the young impressional boy's that they are, as they are growing up. Because our fathers taught us, we feel it incumbent upon us to teach our boys.

Let's look at what many of my male clients have been telling their kids. Firstly, they say that size matters. Boys learn that the size of their penis is a determinant of their sexual potency. The bigger the penis, the manlier you are. What utter, sinful garbage. Sure size matters, but it's most certainly not what should make or break a man's sense of masculinity. A small penis well manipulated can satisfy a woman, and a large penis might be a total waste of time and space. Learn to work with what you have and don't be shy and never apologise for what you have to offer.

And it is true that the larger and thicker the penis, the more chance of satisfying a woman (or a man). But that isn't the only factor to pleasing women. It is the emotional attachment, the intimacy, and the skill with other parts of the body that we bring to the party, which actually matters in such personal and vulnerable times such as these. Penis size is only one part of the mix of sexual satisfaction; the main thing is what a man does with his penis, his hands, his mouth, his fingers and his words. The Japanese have traditionally small penises, but a willing and competent Japanese lover can send a lady through the roof with his abilities. Black men are traditionally supposed to have larger penises (and if you've ever seen a porn film, you'll know that some of them have to be strapped to their knees). But unless the black man is empathetic, loving, supportive and considerate and sensitive to his lover, then he may reach his climax, but will his partner?

The other thing that kids learn (not usually from parents, but from other kids and the exposure to the pornographic material) is that sex is only about penetration. Anything other than penetrative sex is, well, not true sex. I've got news for you; this is wrong. So. Totally. Wrong. There is so much more about love, caring, sex, intimacy and sensuality we need to explore before we even consider the mere idea that penis meets vagina, penis penetrates the vagina, penis 'sneezes orgasm', vagina feels sad and more often than not accumulates resentment. Which will probably not show until after many years of build up?

At least three of my clients in the past six months haven't had penetrative sex in years. Their true intimacy comes from mutual adoration, kissing, fondling, mutual masturbation, and finally – and this is so important – hugging after each has brought the other to a sexual climax using their hands, fingers and mouths; they don't roll over and go to sleep, but instead, lay in each other's arms and hug. That's it, they just hug, hold each other and hug each other and press their bodies together. Sometimes, they would fall asleep like that, and at other times, they'd listen for the other's gentle and rhythmic breathing, kiss each other, and then fall asleep.

Here is another myth that needs to be busted wide open. It's often said that a woman takes a long time to work up to having sex. But that a man is always open to it, in a permanent state of concupiscence, sexual awareness and readiness. It's as if they were walking around with a penis almost full of blood, and waiting, just waiting for the right opportunity to fill to the brim, rise in a throbbing erection, and penetrate. Forgive the expression, gentlemen (and any ladies who are reading this), but that is total BS. Men aren't always ready for sex. Sure, adolescents often have an uncontrollable woodie/stiffie/hard-on, whatever it's referred to these days. But it often happens on a bus going home from school, meaning that the poor kid has to go three stops past his home before his pants return to normal.

But as we get older, more sophisticated and more sexually experienced, it can take a man just as long as a woman to be aroused to have penetrative sex. It's not that the penis doesn't react by filling with blood, but responsibilities and life's disappointments, of all kinds, and the thousand other things which flesh is heir to, will affect a man's ability to become erect.

So let's talk about something, which is called, 'DTF' Yes, it's 'Down To F**k'. As a society, we place too much emphasis on a man's libido, and so the occasional lack of desire can sometimes feel emasculating for some guys. Things like diet, sleep, stress, negative thinking, even hydration will affect anyone's – that is men and women's – performance.

So let me now tell you about one of my male clients. Here is an example of what we should do to teach our kids properly about the mutual responsibilities, and requirements of real empathetic physical intimacy. Now well into his Third Age, this man came to me for weight loss and other health issues. But we became friends, and sometimes met for coffee. During one of our lovely breaks, he told me about his introduction to sex, and how a mature lady had shown him not just what to do for himself, but what a woman seeks from an intimate engagement with a man. Let's call him Guy. Here's the story precisely as he told it to me.

"When I was 17 my then girlfriends Mother, Karen, seduced me. The relationship went on for about 12 months. My parents found out and flipped their lids. Unbeknown to me at the time they confronted Karen and warned her off. When I found out, I was pissed off!

"She was a beautiful woman. One of those rare ones who simply needed sex nearly every day. And let me hazard to add, there is nothing wrong with that.

"That first night of seduction with her is probably still one of the most exciting wonderful things in my memory bank that ever happened to me.

"That evening, I turned up late and drunk to take her daughter Georgette, (my girlfriend at the time) to dinner and the movies. It was a blessing in disguise for me. Georgette was pissed off with me, so she left and went out with our other friends. Clearly I was in deep shit.

"Karen brought me into the house, gave me a good talking too. I was suddenly sick from my early over alcoholic indulgence, I just made the bathroom and threw up. What a bloody mess. So she told me to have a shower and clean up.

"When I came back out, she had coffee for me, and we sat on the lounge and watched TV.

"She must have felt sorry for me, and she seemed to have forgiven me.

"After a while, she moved up close to me and started to caress me. I got the resultant erection, and she began to stroke me.

"Without a word, she stood up, took me by the hand to her bedroom. Undressed both of us and pulled me into bed. I was instructed to lie still and let her have her way with me. She then started to teach me how to pleasure her. This went on for about 3 hours; I was not allowed to penetrate her until she was satisfied I knew what to do and how to please her. It was mind blowing, and being able to pleasure her soon became my main goal over the ensuing 12 months.

"I can recall spending hours performing the most tantalising oral sex, tasting her sweetness, exploring inside that beautiful vagina with my lips, tongue and fingers. It became my particular piece of expertise, and she always marvelled at what she had taught me.

"I was totally in Lust.

"So in effect, I was trained in the art of satisfying my female partner. It's rare that I allow myself to climax or orgasm until I am confident that my partner has experienced my foreplay ritual. It might sound a bit contrived, but time and time again with a new partner, it was clear that most of them had never been treated like this, with respect, with real passion and to make them desperate for the main event to happen".

One of my favourite sayings is, 'Making love to a woman is like spending months and years learning how to play the violin. And once you learn, then you need to use all your skills to play the instrument properly. It's only then that you are rewarded with the sweetest sounding notes'.

If only parents taught their children the lessons that, Guy learned from Karen. She, an older, mature and sexual woman, taught him the skills necessary to live his life within a loving partnership. It's going to be hard for parents to teach their children lessons in such things, like how and where to touch, how to pleasure. So what we need to teach them is how to respect self-love, how to enjoy touching themselves, and bringing themselves to the pleasure we also need to teach them when to say no, and how to learn what their dislikes are. Because once they find out how to please themselves and are open about it, and become more aware, their minds will start to align with their bodies, only then will they be more receptive to other peoples' feelings.

In ancient Greece, that beautiful sexually unrepressed society, there were women called Haterade, who's job it was to teach youngsters all about sex.

Usually, young pubescent boys were taken by their parents to a Hera, who then taught the boy about his body and how to pleasure it, and also showed him how to pleasure and treat a woman. After many lessons, the boy would be returned to his parents, and would then be allowed to marry. Yes, they were a class of prostitute, but a very elevated and superior woman, whose sexual services were rewarded by their rank in society.

Which brings me on to another case study, this time of John and Beth. These are two active and lovely people, married for more than two decades, and desperate for their marriage to continue; but they have a serious problem, and that is one of communication. So let me tell you how things turned out when they came to see me.

John, aged 60 and Beth age 51 have been married for 22 years. They have two sons aged twenty-two and eighteen. Both boys have moved out of the home.

The freedom of no kids in the family home caught John and Beth a bit by surprise; they felt a bit lonely at first, but soon a sense of freedom overcame them, with John hoping for an improved sex life.

Unfortunately, something was missing in their relationship and John's hopes with more time and rooms available in their home. He thought that 'more often' and 'more adventurous' was a given. No?

But the brick wall that had been built between them over the past 15 or 16 years seemed impossible for John to break down or to even change just a little bit.

So now some 12 months since the kids moved out and some failed attempts by John to get Beth to open up, soften and to show some interest in more healthy sexual activities, resulted in John becoming quite sullen in the relationship, feeling hard done by, left out and forgotten. He started playing more golf, spending more time at work and things between he and Beth became more like flatmates.

The old days, they used to have a naughty weekend every two months, and it seemed to be a rule that they would have sex on the first night, typically a Friday night and backing up on Saturday night after going out for a meal and a show.

"God, even if I could go back to that I'd be happy" mused John. "But now we're lucky to get it away once or twice a year. I can't believe I'm going to live like a bleeding Monk for the next two decades. I need some help, what can I do?"

But what I hear from Beth is somehow a different scenario.

"John's recent attempts to have sex now that the kids have gone are just more of the same old, same old.

"Why don't they teach kids at school how to have sex? All John thinks about is rolling on – rolling off in less than 10 minutes (if I'm lucky). He's blown his bolt, satisfied and fell into a deep sleep, with me not even having been warmed up to engage in physical sex. He never showers at night; his beard is too rough, and his foreplay is … well, John's idea of foreplay is grabbing my tits, squeezing them; a few sloppy tongues kisses and then jump aboard. Oh God, preserve me.

"That's what he calls sex, and now we are arguing about it – but how do I tell him he's simply a dud f**k with no idea how a woman's body works?"

My observations were simple, and I had to tell them eventually that the wellbeing of a couple is not taking one another for granted in any aspects of the relationship. John has simply, not kept himself in shape, overweight by about 10 kilograms; his only exercise is golf. He has a larger than average penis, has no trouble in getting and maintaining an erection. But he reckons he knows how to use it.

It seems that 'Wham, bam thank you Ma'am!' is more of his style. He has never engaged in foreplay or tried to have Beth 'hanging off the rafters' desperate for him to sink his huge penis inside her 'cause he's got her so hot and needy from his expert foreplay actions.

Beth goes to the gym five days a week including some Yoga. She is trim, taught and looks great for her age. She is secretly sexually frustrated and has been masturbating more often in the past six months. She has a vibrator and looks forward to John playing golf on Saturdays so she can spend a good couple of hours pleasuring herself – and she has incredible orgasms. "But how can I achieve that with a good-looking man with a beautiful hard penis buried inside me?" she says.

What is the problem here?

John feels let down and upset that Beth won't give him any sex. But obviously, he is clueless.

Beth wants sex, really badly, but considers John simply inept. And she doesn't know how to have an open and frank discussion with him for fear of damaging his ego.

So what is the solution? Simply said, they need help – serious help. And it's not that far away. But they both have to agree to get help from a professional. Luckily enough, they did. I asked Beth to find the strength to open the discussion with John and tell him that, from her point of view, his actions are her problem.

John needs to listen to Beth.

Beth also needs to open up a bit and coax him; help John – but she does need to open the door and let him in, so to speak.

They both came separately as per their request, and after the initial consultation that helped me build an individual profile, I was able to help them out.

I was able to show them how to break down the various barriers to starting healing their relationship.

What John and Beth didn't realise was that if they didn't fix the sexual block between them that the whole relationship will continue to break down and this could lead to an unpleasant, sad and unnecessary breakup.

Beth and John were taking care of themselves by taking seven simple steps to better understanding their personal strengths and weaknesses and that of course as a couple. Of course figuring this out is never easy but the reality of it was that they just couldn't leave things as they were. Both of them urgently require more of and better quality sex. And both have bodies that would respond to the right kind of intimacy. But neither is aware of the problems, which they were causing onto their partner. John was aggrieved; Beth was frustrated.

Both are desirous of a better way of life, but the thing that was missing between them is communication. I listened to John, and then I looked and heard what Beth has to say, and they were miles apart. So I saw it as my job to bring the two of them so close that they could hear each other's problems, and talk them through.

How did I get two people to talk to each other when both of their ears were blocked by years and years of frustration? The solution I suggested was to apply the '7Cs of Intimacy'. This is what I told John and Beth.

The 'C's of Intimacy' are:

1. Communication
2. Care
3. Creative
4. Corporeal
5. Carnal
6. Conflict, and
7. Crisis

Research shows that intimacy is a highly important aspect of any relationship – Yes, even the all-important relationship that is with yourself. And believe it or not, it is vital to your wellbeing. My advice to you and your partner is to stop and ask yourselves. Are you getting any? Are you honestly getting any kind of Intimacy? Remember Intimacy is a contact sport for the soul, not just the body.

When you are beginning to feel hopeless or worthless, I recommend taking a look at the following two aspects and thinking about them for the next week.

COMMUNICATION

a) Learn to say what you mean in the nicest way possible

b) Use "I" or "me" statements, don't ever start any form of communications (even those with yourself) with 'you' or 'you never'. Try these instead, "I have been feeling …" "I've noticed that …" When using these statements, it often softens the delivery of what's about to come. Remember, it's never about what you say; rather it's about how you say it.

CONFLICT

a) When two people come from different upbringings with two completely different sets of morals and emotional understandings decide to make a life together, conflict is going to happen. Each of us comes into a relationship with the various ways of looking at the world, and when these different perceptions clash, we encounter conflict. It isn't about right or wrong; it's about viewpoints and how we see the world.

b) If you continue to meet conflict with defensiveness, you'll find yourselves in a power struggle that fills your relationship with negativity and resentment. If, however, you encounter conflict with willingness and the aim to listen, to actually find out, with empathy for each other, then there's a space for healing and growth to happen.

Creating a well-balanced relationship that covers all of the 'C's' is not an easy feat. It takes hard work and dedication mixed with trust and an understanding that you are two people coming into this relationship with completely different pasts and future expectations. So go easy on yourselves. Have fun and don't punish yourselves for stumbling along the way. How you pick yourselves up is what makes your relationship last in this society we have built, full of demands, expectations and requirements.

The title of this chapter is 'Are men in this alone?' So let me tell you about another client who came to see me, due to his inability to cope with a situation, which had recently occurred, a situation, which was driving him crazy.

Dan was a successful businessman, who'd built up a considerable fortune during his years and years of hard work. He had a large and comfortable house with a spectacular view, a country estate, and a beach house. He and his wife Debbie took regular holidays abroad, and life seemed to be good for them. But only from the outside looking in.

Within the marriage, Dan was deeply unhappy with his sex life. Debbie was a wonderful woman and had been the sort of wife who'd supported him in his business and personal life. Now that their kids were adults and off their hands, she'd taken up golf and the gym four days a week, while Dan went off to work.

Their personal lives were full of socialising, music and entertainment, but when they got home at night, it was the customary twice a month vanilla sex and then good night, and thanks you. Have they not heard that you never say thank you after sex, unless you are paying for it? They use sex as a transactional favour, and that sucks. Now that we are on the subject there a few things you never say after sex. You never mention his mother, or pat his bum and say, that's ok now you can leave. And if sex was better than a root canal, you better find the right time to tell him.

Ok now let's continue with Dan's story.

Dan met Elise through a website where his wealthy friends had told him they'd met spectacular mistresses. Late one night, he'd explored the site, joined, and suddenly Elise turned up. They met one day for coffee, then a couple of days later for lunch, and then they'd spent Friday afternoon in a hotel. And it was the very best sex that Dan had had in his entire life.

He came stronger than he'd ever come before, and even after he'd come, Elise ran a bath and massaged him so that he came again. He felt potent, masculine, powerful all the things he had wanted to feel, but rarely did.

Elise was 41 years old; divorced, tall, with a small tattoo on her shoulder, her one obeisance to Bohemianism; well, that and doing what a friend of hers had done, and joined the website.

She did it because she needed some financial help, but mainly because she wanted to meet a man, and have regular sex … real raunchy sex, not like the 'wham bang thank you ma'am sex', which her divorced husband had given her, when he wasn't drunk.

Dan and Elise met many times that and the following month. He told Debbie that he was particularly busy at work, and the weekends he took away were on business. But things got out of hand between Dan and Elise. He fell in love with her. Head over heels. So much so that he decided to divorce Debbie after eight months of his sexual fling with Elise. Debbie didn't know about it, because he was very circumspect about what he did, and was good at keeping secrets. He went to see his accountant, a friend of many years, and openly discussed his plans. For four hours, the two men drew up best and worst case scenarios for the split.

Dan soon realised that in a divorce court, he'd lose more than half of his assets. Because his wife was a director of his companies, she had a rightful claim to their income and assets. Along with half of his companies, he'd lose the family home and one other property.

Stunned, he drove home, and it took him days to decide on his next move. That was his position when he came to see me, suffering from stress, anxiety, and weight-loss. He just couldn't make up his mind and was suffering.

"I know I'm a bit like a kid who can't choose between one delicious cake and another, but I'm in a terrible state at the moment, and I just don't know what to do".

So he explained to me the details of his problem. It was a serious case of an intellectual, physical, emotional and financial division. With the gorgeous Elise, Dan would spend his life having brilliant regular teeth-clenching sex, a chance to start a brand new life full of adventures and travels to places that Debbie wasn't interested in going. Fun, more intimacy and with more intensity. He was desperate to be with her.

But on the other hand, to leave his wife would mean losing almost everything which he'd worked so hard to acquire, and giving it to Debbie, who, apart from being a good and loyal wife to him and mother to his children, had done nothing to help him build up their assets. He didn't believe she deserved that kind of reward.

I listened to what he said, and I had to fight very hard to keep calm. I wanted to scream at him, "How dare you talk like that about a woman who'd given you her everything throughout her life. Stuck by you through your struggles and helped you to believe in yourself. She has been your rock through thick and thin!"

But I didn't. I remained calm and professional and asked him to take me through the years of his hard work to build his company. He told me about the early years, and I asked him, "So when you got home at night, exhausted, did you have a meal waiting for you? And were the kids bathed and in their PJ's and ready for bed?" He said they were.

And so we went through more and more years, until eventually, and it took the best part of another hour-long session, he could see that Debbie had not only been a partner in everything he'd done, not only been an integral part of his ability to build his fortune and his assets, but that she'd been the loyal one who'd enabled him to become the man he was today.

After two sessions, he accepted that Elise was a wonderful distraction, a novelty which had given him intense pleasure. So I told him to think hard before he made a decision. I brought up the reality that his integrity at work, the way he runs the company, was excellent, so why wouldn't he do that in his life. And because of their shared religious background, he was feeling intense guilt about his affair.

So he continued with the sessions, and he decided that the affair needed come to an end. He came to see me some months later for a follow-up session and told me that he'd fallen back in love with his wife. He also said that he was going to make amends and improve their relationship.

But I still questioned his motives, what was the reason for his sudden spark of love with his wife.

Did he finally understand that his wife was, indeed, an integral part of his growth as a businessman, or did he come to the realisation that the loss of half his fortune was the factor, which had put an end to his affair with Elise?

I don't know. Only time will tell. But for now, he is still with Debbie, who regularly goes to the gym, and has improved her golf handicap; and she's none-the-wiser.

So ask yourself what you'd have done if you were Dan? Split, or Stay?

CHAPTER EIGHT

Human beings are the only species to practice
faithful monogamy ... Yeah right!

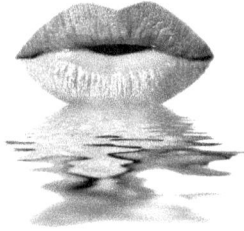

*"I have just learned that penguins are monogamous for
life, which doesn't really surprise me all that much because
they all look exactly alike. It's not like they're going to
meet a better-looking penguin someday."*

Ellen DeGeneres

First, a few relevant definitions. Why? Because in this chapter, you have to know what we mean by what we're saying. And you have to understand the difference between some states of relationships that are being referred to.

So, let's start off with Monogamy. Monogamy means only having one partner in a sexual relationship. A legal contract, such as a marriage certificate, doesn't necessarily have to be part of a monogamous relationship.

Polygamy, on the other hand, is thought to mean having many legal partners. In the religion of Islam, for instance, a man can be married to four women at the same time. Among Mormons, it used to be common to have several wives. Being in a relationship, and having an external sexual relationship with another person, isn't being polygamous.

Polyamory is the state of having several intimate partners at the same time, generally with the knowledge and consent of the other partners. But, in polyamorous relations, there is typically no contractual, religious or other signifiers of permanency.

Adultery is when a partner steps out of a marital situation and has a sexual relationship with another person. Adultery Occurs without the consent of the marital partner.

Celibacy is a state in which a man or woman has no partner and does not have sexual intercourse with another person. 'They often masturbate, to fulfil a physical need. It is the state of abstaining from marriage or any sexual relationships, either willingly or unwillingly.

According to Jake Heppner of distractify.com. Most of us spend very little time having sex as opposed to everything else that we do in life. He found that over a lifetime, the average American will sleep the equivalent of 25 years, work the equivalent of over ten years and have sex an equivalent of a mere 48 days! Sex is a blink in the big picture of relationships and monogamy is not necessarily a reality for everyone.

So what is the reality of monogamy in today's society? This is a 'sexual expression' of offensive consequences to some, and yet an astonishing number of marriages end up in divorce due to infidelity.

That number is 17% and according to FOX news about 70% of men admits to cheating on their wives! Another study found that two out of three women are unaware of their husbands' affairs.

Monogamy is a state, which has been dictated to human beings by religious institutions. From our earliest days in society, we've been told that a man must have a wife in order to procreate. Once they have entered into this institution called 'Marriage' – which is a match made in heaven (Yeah, right! Well at least for the first few years sadly some for only a few months) – neither of them is to have sexual relations with any other person. So, hold on a minute, what happens when we reach "complacency" typically after 2 years of marriage or even worst we reach the "other" annoying phase of the marriage. Say after two to three years for the "C" word (compliancy) and seven, ten or even twenty-five years for the "A" (annoying)? Did you know that cheating typically happens once couples are settled down and start having kids? Their lives are usually more fulfilled in other areas, and the romance starts fading away, they start taking each other, and their marriage for granted and the sex becomes automated.

Well hello? No doubt, there must be someone out there that is obeying the 'rules' placed on us by doctrinarian entities. But can we measure the 'norm' by the exception to the rule?

The bottom line here though is the significance of the major issue. Is monogamy a natural state of affairs? Is it the sort of condition to which human beings were born?

That is something that has been argued by sociologists and philosophers since time began. If you want my opinion (and this is entirely my opinion), I believe that it is crazy to confine yourself to one person for the whole of your adult life. Unless of course you are both part of what I call a team. Meaning, you have reached a stimulated connection not only on a physical and mental level but on an emotional level with your significant other.

Whereby, you are both completely transparent and honest within your relationship and the chosen state of monogamy and the lifestyle that you have selected is a part of who you have decided to become together rather than have it thrust upon you by societies' expectations.

Don't take me wrong, although I don't believe humans are monogamous I do believe in the power of choice and that we are entirely capable to decide for ourselves if we want to be in a monogamous relationship – or not – for that matter. I am very aware that monogamy, in some religions and cultures is of precious value; a highly sought after commodity, but this is quite sporadic in the animal kingdom.

You see, out of the approximately five thousand species of mammals on this earth, only three to five percent are known to committing to a lifelong partner. This group includes beavers, otters, wolves, some bats and foxes and limited hoofed animals. But what is the main difference between humans and mammals? Yes, you guessed right … our brain, our cognitive functions; the biggest issue and controversy would be, are we different in kind or by just a degree to the rest of the animal kingdom? Are we the smartest of them all like Charles Darwin supports or are we a species of our own?

For the most part, we humans can reason. Therefore, we have the capacity to choose what suits us best, with our best interests in mind. Oh, the power of superior intellect!

However, this is a chapter about Monogamy, a permanent relationship between partners, which excludes a sexual relationship with another person. Who are we trying to fool with this concept? All you have to do is go onto some websites.

Ashley Madison claimed to have an international membership of 37.6 million; all of them assured that their use of this service would be 'anonymous', '100% discreet'. With the slogan of 'Life is too short – have an affair' who could resist right?

Don't misinterpret what is being said. Only facts are stated here.

It is my belief that for as long as we can, once we have found the love of our lives, we should marry and do anything in our power not to become a statistic and rather stay married, especially if we want to have children, and yes I mean in a monogamous and committed relationship.

So, if the protections of the rights of children aren't the only reason for marriage, why do we have to be monogamous? Most men … well, 95% want to have experiences with other women apart from their wives. Seventy percent have admitted to it!* And if women were honest with themselves, the same would be true of them, of course for entirely different reasons. It has been proven to me time and time again through meeting and dealing with many clients, that men cheat for the act of sex, while women tend to cheat for more emotionally based reasons. Or at least a vast majority does. This is what is happening in our society today. We are just not talking about it.

The aim of this book is not to scare you but to bring awareness. We have to talk openly and transparently about the taboos in our society so that the constant misunderstandings and miscommunications no longer occur. We must stop being the cause of psychologically disturbed children. After all, it's our children who will become society's leaders in the years to come and if they don't have a bedrock of understanding societal norms, then how can they become the sort of people that the younger generations will want to follow?

For my research, and to have an understanding of both men and women's perspectives and desires while writing this book, I became a member of an adult's only dating site. To protect the people I have met from this site I will not share any information about which dating site. For the men and women who advertise their availability on this website, they are looking for one sure thing … a designer relationship, with the mutual understanding, that there is a basis of physical intimacy. And sure, it might have become a situation where the man was expected to be generous with the lady, and pamper her, by gifting her with presents, trips and other incentives, with the expectation of a physically intimate relationship in return. This site is not a prostitution site. Each party has the inalienable right to reject somebody he or she doesn't want.

So I went onto this site and became a member to see the sorts of men who were on there, and what they wanted. It intrigued me to find out what it was exactly that these people wanted and why they were looking, as in most cases they were still in fact married?

I didn't have to go very far, as the amazing thing was that just by reading some of their profiles, I was exposed to a whole new world in the dating scene. In almost no instance did the man explicitly say that he wanted sex. A large percentage said that they wanted a relationship with a woman, well, more like a 'situation' with someone other than his wife. Someone who would be sweet, loving, kind, thoughtful, intimate, passionate, erotic ... all the things which his wife could have been, but in most cases wasn't or might have been in the early stages of their relationship, but who no longer fulfils this role.

The women requested similar, yet different things. Most women on the site didn't want a 'relationship' they wanted excitement, somebody to care for them, someone to pamper them and show them the life they'd hoped their husbands would provide. Again this is exactly why perhaps they were attracted to their husbands, to begin with, in the early stages, and chose them to be the father of their children, but somewhere along the way that all went pear shaped.

On the surface, the women on this site came across as gold-diggers, but when you stripped away the façade that this web site provided, it was apparent that the men and females wanted the same thing. Something that they were currently lacking! That is affection, intimacy, pampering, consideration, an individual connection and of course a sense of importance and being made to feel central to another person's life.

To be told that they were special, to be noticed and reminded that they were more than just a provider, father, a chef or a mother. They wanted to feel alive in a physical and more intimate way. Holding hands, kissing and being made to feel like the lover that they once felt they were! My question is unless you declare yourself as polyamorous why can't this be the societal norm? Or perhaps even be able to open up to expressing the way you feel, maybe even staging a fantasy with our wife or husband?

Accompanying this book in our limited edition *Intimacy Kits* is an enclosed XXX guide with some great ideas games and toys to re-engage with your significant other gently. I encourage you to role-play to find your innermost erotic sensual self and show it off to your loved one. Spice things up. I dare you!

In the meantime read on to see what exactly men and women are looking for when they think they have nothing to lose!

Here are some examples of the sorts of profiles which I found on the website ...

"... I want someone who can show me things they have never experienced before. I love the adventure of life and am looking for someone to share that with. I want to have and connect with someone where we can just be ourselves. Someone who can have a laugh with me at times but can be serious also (but mostly let's just have fun!) Let's try new and novel hedonistic adventures together. Offer me something to make me laugh, capture my imagination, engage my curiosity and inspire my desire".

"... What I'm Looking for is a woman who understands intimacies of all kinds, it is what all men want and especially a lady who enjoys being intimate".

Ladies that are reading this book are we listening to these comments?

"... There is no limit to what life and this amazing world can offer us if we are open to the possibilities. I want to experience it all. I'm caring, gentle but also robust and confident. Let's just let it unfold and see where it takes us. I'm single for the first time in a very long time and interested to explore life, fun, passion and sensuality. But mostly I miss the intimacy, which I once enjoyed, and which disappeared when we had kids".

"... I am seeking a person who enjoys romance, good company and is confident by nature. She must be a good conversationalist, enjoy surprises and lives life to the full. Enjoys living for the now rather than worrying about tomorrow. Open-minded and adventurous are key traits together with a sense of humour. Seeking a cheeky, uninhibited woman who loves sensuality, bedroom adventures and pampering ..."

"... Fun, witty, humorous and someone authentic in an arrangement. Be you, not you that you envisage society thinks you should be. Explore in a safe, discreet environment and then step back into your world with just a cheeky grin ..."

"... Yes, I desire intimacy from this relationship, but also much more; I want fun and companionship to an extent! Let's start out small and see where we go! You'll need to be challenging and resourceful. During the time we're together, I'd like you to be along ON the ride, rather that be taken for a ride ...!"

"... I'm looking for one particular, attractive woman whose eyes are wide open, enjoys and appreciates all life has to offer and wants an exclusive relationship with a fun, old friend, lover and mentor. If you're charming and beautiful (inside & out), love to smile & laugh, are sweet, sensual, healthy and appreciate the great conversation and a mature man, then maybe we'll have found our match in one another. If so, whatever lights us up, let's explore the possibilities ..."

Now, what is it that the ladies are seeking from such an arrangement? For me to find out, I asked a male friend to join the site, and do precisely what I'd done so that we could discover the other side of the coin.

From his observations, most of them wanted to be controlled. We are not going to judge the site on the exceptions so please note that although we didn't dive into the search misleading anyone, generally speaking we found that to females of all ages and colours it was a search for somebody who'll look after them financially, culturally, socially and then finally it was to have the ability to fulfill the man's fantasies and desires, this may be surprising for some, but it is true, a lot of women desire the ability to satisfy their lover. Is this wrong? Well, according to society's judgmental rules and regulations, it is incorrect.

In my belief, nothing is right or wrong. It just is. We are all different and require different things to be happy and healthy individuals.

Sure, they'll have sex with a man they'll meet on this website, but unlike a prostitute who has to service any and every man who walks through the door, these individuals can choose to have a relationship with somebody or not. It is obligation free. And it's the same with other dating and adult websites. That's the advantage of this fast-growing aspect of the XXX side of the Internet. It's giving women who need support and companionship, the right to choose, the right to be more in control.

And control is one of the aspects which is most prominent on this dating website I joined. The women who offered themselves to these 'situations' would choose the right mate, and once chosen, the women wanted to be 'looked after'. They wanted the right sides of a normal marital relationship, companionship, intimacy, eroticism and romance.

Here are some of the responses from ladies, and what they sought after …

"… You're intelligent, funny and not an asshole. You take pride in what you've achieved in your life and a non-smoker. I'll find you sexy if you're shy and introverted, or if you're straight to the point and not interested in fluff. You understand that mutual attraction and chemistry is needed to make this kind of arrangement benefit us both …"

"… I seek an open/liberal minded individual to compliment my existing interests/activities. One who could appreciate & respect an independent ladies alternative private lifestyle & be of financial assistance to such activities. I am in a middle management position with my career to a large corporation at this stage of life & looking to expand my personal & professional pursuits with an understanding person male/female. I do not seek an emotional relationship but do seek an ongoing permanent arrangement".

"… I'm drama free and easy going … that said I'm no push over and respect for you and your time is equal to respect for me and my time … read on if genuine … I'm not young so if you are looking for an immature girl skip my profile, but with age comes confidence and experience … ideally looking for either casual meeting with potential for something more regular if the connection is right a devoted lady for the right man for the right arrangement".

So what does this mean in the scheme of things? Well, try this for size.

It is a concept that I am quite fond of. I have come up with this, as I believe this is the answer to keeping a relationship new, fresh and everlasting.

For every relationship that follows our initial attempt – failed Marriage – should have a used by date of two years.

Yes, you read that correctly. Two years.

After two years, we tend to take each other for granted. We become set in our ways. This leads to the inevitable feeling of mutual complacency, and there is a high risk of boredom creeping in.

What happens after the two-year expiry you ask?

After two years in the relationship, I think that both partners should be completely free to say, "I want to explore other relationships. You can either join me or let me fly solo for a while".

Now I know it is not that simple. This kind of scenario I just painted could cause a lot of pain and suffering to both adults involved. That is not fun for anyone.

But on the other hand when we are young and sign up to a long marriage or relationship 'contract' we erroneously presume that with it; we sign up for a lifetime of sexual satisfaction … I guess you already found out that that is far but very far from the truth and you and I know that nothing lasts an eternity but monogamy, treated with respect and helped with some ingenuity, and the sex appeal can be very much kept alive as we grow older together.

I think that after 2 years in our relationship we should reevaluate it, and sign an 'emotional agreement' – yes don't close the book yet, the best is yet to come; hear me out here – before that, we sit down with our partner and chat about our most intimate feelings we are having or wishing we did have, we make a list of the strengths and flaws of the relationship's performance up to the point we are at. This is not to be taken lightly be either partner. It is to be a process that should take a few weekends to complete. It is essential to be treated as a relationship contract so to speak. Due diligence is necessary to decide if continuing the relationship, and signing up for another two years, is what both partners want.

INTIMACY IS A CONTACT SPORT FOR THE SOUL

The process of making love or having sex with a long-term partner is like making art and Intimate is your brush, hands or the gadgets you need. The secrete for a lasting and fulfilling relationship is to make "ART FUN" so let's explore some of the MUST HAVE tools.

Physical Intimacy

The all important sex, how do you feel before and after, what do you like before and after, how and where do you like to be touched, do certain things make you feel uncomfortable, what do you like to do or not do to your partner, do you have any fantasies that you would like to experiment with, name the pros and cons and openly discuss all of this with your partner.

Communication Intimacy: Do you leave notes for one another? Do you send texts or make phone calls? Maybe you used to leave sweet notes for one another but are not doing it anymore, and this is something that you miss and would like to re-introduce? Are you ignoring each other?

Do you feel that you truly communicate? And not just the housekeeping, small talk. But do you share your likes and dislikes often enough, so you know what the other is feeling about everything? Do you feel that you are 'hearing' what the other person is telling you or just being 'heard'? Perhaps you are not really 'listening' to one another? Do you stop, acknowledge and understand what you are communicating to each other or do you just ass-u-me and fill in the blanks for yourself?

Conflict Intimacy

This one is a big one, so make sure you build up solid grounds on this one. Ask yourselves, what irritates you about the other person's behaviour?

Is there anything she/he can do to help you feeling valued? What causes conflict in the relationship according to you, perhaps things that you have been bottling up or don't have the courage to bring up in conversation to avoid the conflict that ensues? How does each of you deal with conflict? Does one of you bottle it up and keep quiet and the other unleash? Do you feel like your partner reciprocates within the relationship?

Parental Intimacy (If you have kids together)

This is also a huge subject and perhaps it deserves a chapter on its own, but let me say this. Before you got married you probably spoke of having children and those children didn't ask you to bring them into this world. So from the moment you thought about and decided to have them, it is your obligation to show them the utmost respect, to show them your unconditional love and be there for them when they need you. On a personal level, things might have changed between you and your partner but one thing will never change, and that is that you are both parents to a child or your children. So you will need to drop your ego, your criticism of and from your partner, you will have to put up with the fact that he/she might be involved in your life, for the rest of your life. One part of your relationship will change, and that is the very essence of being parents so I would strongly suggest you learn very soon to make peace with this and learn the rules of Parental Intimacy.

Ok, let's go back to our list, the one you will have to do every two years.

After you finish the list, I ask that you place a number from one to ten. Ten being the worst you feel about how this particular thing is affecting you in your relationship.

The list shouldn't be longer than a page, but if you find yourself writing and can't stop, you might need to seek the assistance of a third party 'mediator'. Pick someone who doesn't know either of you.

Once you have the 'Strengths and the Flaws List' with the number next to each subject matter, you will add the total for each column

E.g. Strengths list = 9 points and Flaws List = 7 points this will give you a magnificent idea on the things you need to work on and help you to add value to the relationship that you currently have. It also shows where you and your partner have your priorities set and this can be the very essence of some compromises needing to be made. My suggestion then is to work on the 'flaws' and discuss them. Notice that I said 'discuss' them not argue over them. This is where I would usually say to my clients, there is no right or wrong here, there just is! What you and your partner are feeling is not the right or wrong way to feel. It is just the way that you both feel. There is no point telling them that they shouldn't feel a certain way. Instead, understand that this is just how they feel.

What will that mean for the children? Well, it doesn't mean that a loving couple, married or living together will have to split up. They can decide to stay together if they want to and if they feel that this relationship is something worth continuing. I'm sure that almost all of them will decide this. But what this exercise will do, is put pressure on the relationship ... a positive pressure, which, will force each person in the relationship to analyse themselves and think about what he or she needs to do to keep their partner interested and committed. As I mentioned earlier, after two years people begin to take each other for granted, falling into a routine and a pattern of comfort. They don't worry about the way they look so much or the way they smell, if they did or did not change the bed linen after a week, maybe they have put on weight, or they just don't touch anymore the way they used to as they have become all too familiar with one another. Of course, there is nothing wrong with this. It is just a state of comfort, but and I do mean but, is it by losing ourselves in the mundane world of mediocre relationships that we also begin to lose the spark of what a good and healthy relationship could bring.

This gentle but serious pressure will have the effect of revitalising the connection, of refreshing it. Of forcing both partners to think about the relationship from the other's perspective. Am I sexy enough? Am I giving enough? Am I doing what my partner expects? Am I letting myself go? Am I putting on a bit too much weight, or are we losing the delicacy that we had when we first met and found so attractive in each other? Are we paying each other enough attention? Are we treating each other as 'husband' and 'wife' instead of 'mother' and 'father'? If the answer is 'no', then there is plenty of room for improvement. If the answer is 'yes', then the couple will in most instances stay together, but only with improvements, changes, communication and constant refreshment ... every two years or so!

Holding this 'Sword of Damocles' over the heads of their partners will stop the complacency, and will force them to bring back that former condition and vigour that was enjoyed earlier in the relationship. It will refresh the ideas, instincts, lusts, affections, eroticisms, and all the other aspects of that first flush of desire which brought them together. Love doesn't end because we are growing older love gets chipped away because we forget how to take care of each other's needs and assume that all is ok and begin taking each other for granted. And we know what happens when you 'ass-u-me'; it makes an ASS of U and ME. By stopping and listening to each other's needs we reveal something exquisite which is the very essence of our soul, the deepest desires and the core values that make us who we really are. Together we can evolve and elevate each other with respect and unconditional love without having to suppress or deny that inner voice of yours.

I'll bet that if husbands and wives were honest, most would say that after seven or ten years, they just got bored, that love flew out the window. But it didn't. It just needed to be dusted off, refreshed, and given a new coat of paint, at least once every two years. That's why I think that all relationships need a used by date of two years.

Now, am I advocating that all relationships should part after two years? Of course not ... I'm saying that every two years, they need to be reviewed and renewed. Couples have to sit down, talk openly and honestly and transparently about the good, the bad, the happy and the unhappy, and it needs to be a conversation about not just the social, emotional and cultural aspects of the relationship, but the physical aspects too.

Is the connection working for both of us? Am I happy with the way you kiss me, touch me, put your hands on my body? Are you sexually satisfying me? Are we making love enough, too much, or is it becoming too boring, mediocre, and ordinary? And all of this has to be in a non-threatening atmosphere. Comments are not, under any circumstances to be used in the future against the other. These are observations and critiques not ever to be thought of as direct criticisms.

So how do we keep a long-term relationship together? If monogamy is arguably the best state of a relationship for a couple and their children, then is there a way of ensuring that the relationship remains intact, to the satisfaction of both parties? Ever heard of the 'Game Theory'? This is the study of the way in which conflict and cooperation works between intelligent adults. Well, why not bring a bit of game theory, or perhaps some simple games, into a marriage?

Here are some precious reasons why should we aim for a healthy, transparent monogamous steady relationship:

Our children this will provide them with the best stability possible, as children should be protected until they can understand the real complexities that make up the relationships that surround them.

But there's a more important reason, and that is to assure our kids that the 'parental intimacy' is there for them to access at any time whether or not they all live as a united entity under the same roof.

After a certain age, kids can find themselves protected by many different arrangements; at school, through work, unions, and friendships, but it is imperative, as parents, to make the children your absolute number one priority.

Even in the unhappy followings of a divorce, there are ways for a divorcing husband and wife to work around this and to show the kids that your love for them is undivided, even if the marriage is now fractured. Parents need to learn about parental intimacy so that this understanding and acceptance can be passed down through to their children.

Unconditional Love the kind of love that will give us strength and help us support each other with the complex dimensions of our physical, emotional, spiritual and mental bodies, if women tend to cheat for emotional satisfaction and men cheat more from sexual motivation what is this telling us?

CONCLUSION

Man's mind once stretched by a new idea,
never regains its original dimensions

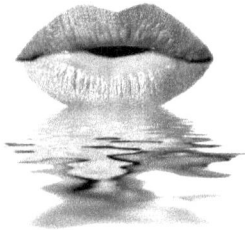

*"The elevator to success is out of order. You'll have to
use the stairs … ONE STEP AT A TIME."*
Joe Girard

The Chinese leader, Mao Zedong, once said that 'a journey of a thousand leagues begins with a single step'.

Wellness, lifestyle and other fitness issues, have never been so essential to the health, well being, and longevity of people. We live in an increasingly polluted and incredibly frenetic world. Fast foods have replaced meals, cars have replaced legs, and television has replaced social and family interactions.

We're overeating, under-exercised, and increasingly frustrated. We're living longer due to good medicine, but enjoying it less as our sedentary lives cause our bodies frequently to suffer diseases and ailments which are the slings and arrows of outrageous fortune.

Which is why this book has been written. Remember that a journey, no matter how long, has, to begin with, a single step. And that's precisely what I've been trying to demonstrate to you. Most lifestyle coaches put their clients on a diet, exercise and wellness routine which is doomed to failure, because it's too much, too quickly, and too different from the way their clients have lived their lives.

My approach, as you'll have seen in this book, is the step-by-step approach. You've been led gently along a road which is pleasant, easy to tread, and simple to accommodate in your normal lifestyle. And after those first steps, when the actions become routine, you'll have already started to incorporate them into your daily life, and you'll already be feeling lots better.

Over the course of reading this book, you were introduced to some of the most interesting people I have had the privilege of working with, people who have helped to shape my understanding of how we humans behave. So much of our behaviour is mitigated by the relationships we form, initially as children, and then as adults when we fall in lust or love or create the partnerships as adults, which lead to a fuller and more satisfying life. These relationships can be monogamous or polyamorous, provided what is done is consensual.

These couples, have been guided by me, but, as in 'Plato's Academy', the teacher learns along with the students, and so my knowledge and expertise as a Wellbeing and Lifestyle Coach have expanded. My clients have helped me to understand the importance of committing to a high level of health and well-being and ensuring that above all else, we as individuals are responsible for our own happiness in our various health and relationship quests. I have compiled this book to pass on my many learned and less successful attempts at achieving a state of balance within my relationships, social life and work life. It is a wish of mine to teach as many people as I can and to open their eyes to seeing life through a new set of eyes so that they can understand and accept that which previously, they may be inclined to judge and perhaps condemn.

You met a couple who for the first time in their marriage were introduced to the inner child of their beloved. Over a phone conversation in the middle of an airport! Here you learnt the importance of knowing who you are and what you need to have you so that your desires can be met at all levels within a relationship. Whether it be mentally or physically.

John and Margaret were next, who were experiencing a lack of intimacy within their marriage; it was so severe that it led, slowly but inexorably to dissatisfaction and all because of a breakdown in communication. This, unfortunately, led Margaret to stray from their marriage and seek an extra martial affair.

Oscar and Lucy were next. It was a lack of rest and sleep on Oscar's part which led to the couple sleeping in different rooms by the time they had come to seek my guidance. You slowly learnt that with a new approach to their health and lifestyle choices, Oscar and Lucy were able to reignite that divine passion and romance in their relationship. All it took was a change in habits when it came to their Nutrition, Sleep and Stressors. In this chapter, we learned that sugar hides behind 61 different names, but merely by eliminating this one toxin, this insidious but ubiquitous poison, we can change our moods, sleep patterns, weight control issues and mindset. It was this positive approach which led to a much happier and healthier state of marriage for these two. Yes, unfortunately, for Lucy and Oscar, it needed to get a lot worse before it could get better. But for you, it doesn't have to be this way at all. I have armed you with basic tools for you to recognise these situations surfacing within your current or future relationships before they get out of hand.

You were introduced to the concept of Intimacy in a variety of ways; Physical, Communication, Conflict, Parental, Carnal and Caring. And that life and love are more than just sex that the majority of intimacies, which we experience, doesn't require or even lead to sex. Rather, that the intimacies we do come by are more than sex, and that sex itself is more than just the physical act.

As a couple, it is important to be open to exploring someone else's thoughts and desires and being able to open yourself up to them in return. This nurturing act is an important ingredient in growing together in strength as a couple.

You need to open up to your own vulnerability. This could potentially mean creating a balance within yourself to have the courage and motivations to be able to, with confidence, confide in your partner. This is a task that is often much harder than what we perceive and takes a lot of time and patience for both parties. But with the right environment and exposure to the relationship, both individuals can flourish and indeed see a whole new side to their relationship together. Opening this door brings with it vast and endless possibilities to be further explored.

The question was asked: Are we by nature monogamous or polyamorous?

We delved a little deeper into this topic, and I showed you why I don't believe that we, as a human race, are in fact monogamous. Of course we do have the power of choice, as we are intelligent beings and can think for ourselves, so it is my belief that rather than have thrust upon us this pressure to be confined to a monogamous relationship for the rest of our lives, as society has so kindly done to us all, we can choose to be in one, two or more relationships. But the key is openness and honesty. If your heart is in a polyamorous relationship, then be honest tell both (or more) partners where your heart is, rather than been deceiving. With all the stresses, tensions and guilt that this generates.you all will benefit from a transparent and honest relationship/s.

I believe that it should not be frowned upon or judged harshly if we decide that monogamy is not for us. The differences between men and women were brought to your attention and why it is difficult to say that we are in fact a monogamous species and why so many of us struggle to come to terms with these expectations which are put on us from such a young age.

And to assist further with this concept, I brought to light the concept of a two-year contract relationship whereby every two years both parties are to sit down with one another and discuss their relationship. What is working for them and what isn't, what they like and what they don't like. And how they feel that they can improve their relationship. What takes place needs to be a mature and understanding conversation between two adults. Being able to express themselves in such a scenario, knowing that the partner can put their hand up and request time out from the relationship, will put a healthy amount of pressure on both parties to try that little bit harder at making their significant other feel wanted, desired, appreciated and special. Because as we read earlier in some quotes from my online dating site research, this is a common underlying factor which most of us adults crave within a relationship.

After reading this book, I hope that you have a new-found respect for your partner, friends, parents and your future relationships. And that you can enter into scenarios with a fresher and more open-minded outlook. These aren't necessarily easy things to accomplish in the short term. That's why I began by quoting Chairman Mao … a long journey begins with one short step.

I've welcomed you onto the path I've trodden in my personal life. I hope that you've enjoyed travelling some distance upon this path and that you've made it your own.

But one thing you have to believe, is that you are NOT alone on this path. I and my colleagues are here for you. You have my email address; you have my website; and, without putting too fine a point on it, you have me.

In Health and Wellness
Patricia Maris

To contact Patricia please scan here.

REFERENCES

Every reasonable effort has been made to contact copyright holders of material reproduced in this book. If any have inadvertently been overlooked the publishers would be glad to hear from them and make useful in future editions, any errors or omissions brought to their attention.

Jane Austen – A quote from Sense and Sensibility. http://www.goodreads.com/quotes/288060-it-is-not-time-or-opportunity-that-is-to-determine

La Belle Dame Sans Merci. http://www.shmoop.com/la-belle-dame-sans-merci/poem-text.html

ADHD Autoimmune disorders have also been implicated in triggering ADHD-like symptoms in susceptible patients. http://www.medscape.com/viewarticle/495640_3

Powerful Sculpture at Burning Man shows Inner Child Trapped Inside Adult Body. http://www.boredpanda.com/burning-man-festival-adults-babies-love-aleksandr-milov-ukraine/

ADD, ADHD. http://www.helpguide.org/articles/add-adhd/attention-deficit-disorder-adhd-in-children.htm

> Myth: Medication is the best treatment option for ADHD. Fact: Medication is often prescribed for attention deficit disorder, but it might not be the best choice for your child. Effective treatment for ADHD also includes education, behaviour therapy, support at home and school, exercise, and proper nutrition.

People (1964 Song) composed by Jule Styne with lyrics by Bob Merrill. https://en.wikipedia.org/wiki/People_(1964_song)

enigma7 – E7Kaizen –https://enigma7.com.au/e7-products-and-services/

> In Japanese, 'Kaizen' is a practice for continuous improvement. At enigma7 we believe that our online programme will give you the tools to strive for a better YOU,

allowing you to improve at your pace while helping you build a stronger wellness foundation.

Physical Intimacy. http://www.healthyplace.com/relationships/intimate-relationships/what-is-physical-intimacy/

Sexuality Dysfunction in the elderly: age or disease? 20 Dec 2005. http://www.nature.com/ijir/journal/v17/n1s/full/3901429a.html

A Cross-National Study of Subjective Sexual Well-Being Among Older Women and Men: Findings From the Global Study of Sexual Attitudes and Behaviours. http://link.springer.com/article/10.1007/s10508-005-9005-3

Using medical treatments to help enjoy sexual activity. http://www.nature.com/ijir/journal/v17/n1s/full/3901429a.html

Edward O. Laumann. https://sociology.uchicago.edu/directory/edward-o-laumann

$100 Billion Industry. http://www.nbcnews.com/business/business-news/porn-industry-feeling-upbeat-about-2014-n9076

Moving Intimacy into the Fridge seminar. http://www.bringintimacyback.com

Metabolic Typing Advice. http://healthexcel.com/public/Advanced.html

To find out what we can do for you follow this link and sign up – Your advisor name is Patricia Maris, and the Advisor Cert # is PM487

Real Relationships. http://www.apa.org/monitor/2014/04/pornography.aspx

Dr. Edward Group DC, NP, DACBN, DCBCN, DABFM Published on March 6, 2013, Last Updated on January 22, 2015. http://www.globalhealingcenter.com/natural-health/9-reasons-exercise-best-medicine/

There is no debate; regular exercise is vital for maintaining health and wellness.

Women's Health Easy Orgasm Book. https://books.google.com.au/
books?id=_FDbCQAAQBAJ&pg=PT94&lpg=PT94&dq=Italian+
researchers+put+a+small+group+of+obese+women+with+sexual+
complaints&source=bl&ots=ArXH62CSyk&sig=Y0xUJFzSqZ1Z
hSg3a098sFqONYM&hl=en&sa=X&ved=0ahUKEwiWopGVw4
bQAhVBRJQKHYlfCB4Q6AEIGzAA#v=onepage&q=Italian%20
researchers%20put%20a%20small%20group%20of%20obese%-
20women%20with%20sexual%20complaints&f=false

https://www.agingcare.com/articles/loneliness-in-the-
elderly-151549.htm

Here are all the ways sleep deprivation is killing your sex life.
http://fusion.net/story/105433/here-are-all-the-ways-sleep-
deprivation-is-killing-your-sex-life/

Living along stats. http://www.abs.gov.au/ausstats/abs@.nsf/
Latestproducts/3236.0Main%20Features62011%20to%20
2036?opendocument&tabname=Summary&prodno=3236.0&iss
ue=2011%20to%202036&num=&view=

http://www.aoa.acl.gov/aging_statistics/profile/2014/2.aspx

Together but Still Lonely. https://www.psychologytoday.com/blog/
the-squeaky-wheel/201306/together-still-lonely

The 7 C's in Intimacy. https://enigma7.com.au/7-cs-intimacy/

The Telegraph – All men watch porn, scientist find. http://www.
telegraph.co.uk/women/sex/6709646/All-men-watch-porn-
scientists-find.html

The Lost City of Pompeii. http://io9.gizmodo.com/5825459/the-
roman-city-of-pompeii-pictures-of-a-lost-world-frozen-in-time

*75% Women either have never had an orgasm or rarely have an
orgasm.* http://abcnews.go.com/Health/ReproductiveHealth/sex-
study-female-orgasm-eludes-majority-women/story?id=8485289

Louise Willy considered the first erotic film in 1899.
http://www.thefrisky.com/photos/6-pioneering-female-porn-stars/
porn_pioneers_louise_willy/

'Hysteria' and the Strange History of Vibrators'.
https://www.psychologytoday.com/blog/all-about-sex/201303/
hysteria-and-the-strange-history-vibrators

The Kama Sutra: Beyond the Sex.
http://www.hinduhumanrights.info/the-kama-sutra-beyond-the-sex/

http://abcnews.go.com/Health/ReproductiveHealth/sex-study-
female-orgasm-eludes-majority-women/story?id=8485289

Jake Heppner. 30 surprising facts about how we spend our time.
http://distractify.com/old-school/2015/01/07/astounding-facts-
about-how-we-actually-spend-our-time-1197818577

FOX news. How to move on after your partner cheated or lied.
http://magazine.foxnews.com/love/cheating-statistics-do-men-
cheat-more-women

*Cancer is not a reductionist phenomenon. Understanding
Reductionist vs. Holistic Thinking.*
https://weilerpsiblog.wordpress.com/2012/01/05/understanding-
reductionist-vs-holistic-thinking/

The Guardian. Life After the Ashley Madison affair.
https://www.theguardian.com/technology/2016/feb/28/what-
happened-after-ashley-madison-was-hacked

Game theory. https://en.wikipedia.org/wiki/Game_theory

Divorce Rates Around The World. The USA 53% – Australia 43%
in 2010. http://www.businessinsider.com.au/map-divorce-rates-
around-the-world-2014-5

TITLES TO WATCH OUT FOR

Born With a Manual

Kids today are entering a world so entirely different from anything, which any previous generation has ever experienced. The internet, social media, 2-4-3-6-5 news, visual images everywhere which would once have had people jailed, it's all there. And our kids are taking it all in with gusto and glee which makes their parents' heads spin. This book is dedicated to all children entering into one of the most difficult ages of their lives and yet an age full of energy and indecisions ... But also an impeccable inherited ability to self-sabotage.

The Naked Intimacy

Our parents and grandparents used to be ashamed of nudity, nakedness, sexuality, lust and gratification. 'Parental Intimacy' is all about the exposure of the body, the mind and the soul. In other words TRANSPARENCY. For some, it can be enlightening, liberating and delightful. For others, it can be confronting, affronting and condemnatory. *The Naked Intimacy* is about 'Parental Intimacy' the intimacy, which every parent should be obligated to assume before we even graduate with such a privileged title. Parents!

The Unfinished Animal

Physical, sexual and emotional abuse is more prevalent today than ever before. Whether there's more of it, or whether people are no longer hiding, but coming forward to report it to the authorities, is something which is still being determined. Abuse is a destructive cycle, which takes strength, determination and courage to break. It often means a splitting of a relationship, and can lead to further hatred, but not reporting it and putting a stop to it can result in irreparable damage ... even death. *The Unfinished Animal* is based on a true story, the life after sexual emotional and physical abuse, of a young woman looking for redemption and trying to figure out what is next in life.

Beyond Age Beyond Colour Beyond Gender

We live in a youth culture that has inherited emotional pain amongst other things. Most of our advertising, media, communications and entertainment is created by, directed at and consumed by the young. BUT the world is growing older. We're reaching ages in life never before attained. It's not uncommon for hale and hearty men and women to be working, doing sports and enjoying life in their mid-80s and beyond. So this is a book dedicated to those of us who have put family cares and responsibilities behind us, and are looking forward to a full and active life without the pressures of youth or the silliness of 'What if'! It's for when the colour of your skin does not match the colour of your organs when your chronological age has nothing to do with the state of your mind, and when the power of love has nothing to do with your genitalia.

OUR SOCIAL MEDIA LINKS

FACE BOOK

LINKEDIN

TWITTER

INSTAGRAM

www.ingramcontent.com/pod-product-compliance
Lightning Source LLC
Chambersburg PA
CBHW071125280326
41935CB00010B/1122